Intercollegiate MRCS
Part A: SBAs and EMQs

Mock papers with comprehensive answers

CHARLOTTE DUNFORD
MBBS BSc (Hons) MRCS
Core Surgical Trainee, Oxford Deanery

SARAH WALDMAN
MA (Cantab) MBBChir MRCS
Academic Clinical Fellow in General Surgery, Oxford Deanery

ZOE BARBER
MA (Oxon) BM BCh MRCS
Core Surgical Trainee, Oxford Deanery

Foreword by

(EMERITUS) PROFESSOR JOHN MORRIS
MD, MA, FMed Sci
Intercollegiate MRCS Examiner
Department of Physiology, Anatomy & Genetics, University of Oxford

Radcliffe Publishing
London • New York

Radcliffe Publishing Ltd
33–41 Dallington Street
London
EC1V 0BB
United Kingdom

www.radcliffehealth.com

British Library Cataloguing in Publication Data

A catalogue record for this book is available from the British Library.

ISBN-13: 978 190891 154 4

The paper used for the text pages of this book is FSC® certified. FSC (The Forest Stewardship Council®) is an international network to promote responsible management of the world's forests.

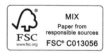

Typeset by Darkriver Design, Auckland, New Zealand
Printed and bound by TJI Digital, Padstow, Cornwall, UK

Contents

MRCS Part A Paper 2 Answers   184

Foreword

The format of the Intercollegiate MRCS Part A examination has now become established. From September 2012 Part A Paper 1 will consist of 135 single best answer questions, whereas Part A Paper 2 will consist of 135 themed extended-match or single best answer questions, each to be completed in 2 hours. Students preparing for the examination will be well advised to practise for this type of examination, and this is just the book to help them. Charlotte Dunford, Sarah Waldman and Zoe Barber are all trainee surgeons who have used their experience of sitting and passing the examination for the benefit of those coming after them. They have carefully adjusted the question topics to reflect the balance in the exam, but sensibly provided two sets of five practice papers, each with a reduced number of questions to be completed in 45 minutes. As someone who, for many years, has helped trainees prepare for the exam and also acted as an examiner, I would recommend anyone preparing for MRCS Part A to work their way through these mock papers. Getting the answers right will boost their confidence and, with a little more work, they will learn from any mistakes.

(Emeritus) Professor John Morris MD, MA, FMed Sci
Intercollegiate MRCS Examiner
Department of Physiology, Anatomy & Genetics
University of Oxford
March 2013

Preface

This is a practice-question book designed as an aid to postgraduate MRCS Part A revision, but can also be used by undergraduate students sitting surgical finals. It consists of 10 mock revision papers, each with 50 questions. It has been written by surgical trainees who have recently completed the MRCS examination and is designed in accordance with 2012 Royal College of Surgeons of England guidance. The 2012 guidelines are very precise regarding how each paper is broken down and weighted to each theme, topic and sub-specialty. We have compiled mock revision papers to reflect this, providing you, the student, with an up-to-date revision guide.

Each question not only reflects core knowledge, as outlined in the Royal College of Surgeons of England MRCS syllabus, but also draws on our experience as junior surgical trainees. As such, each question is written to reflect not only the level of knowledge needed but also the application of that knowledge, both of which are required to complete the written MRCS examination. The questions range from simple knowledge recall of essential facts to more complex questions requiring synthesis of the information presented in the question before making a decision on further management. In our experience, this book accurately reflects the level of questioning seen in the MRCS examinations.

Answers are included and written clearly and concisely. In writing these, we have assumed a certain level of surgical knowledge (i.e. completion of surgical final examinations at undergraduate level). While this should be adequate in the physiology and pathology explanations, for the most part, anatomy is poorly grasped at an undergraduate level, so you may need a reference book to further explain and help you visualise key anatomy points that are mentioned frequently in the examination. The questions cover a broad range of topics but not all – this book is designed to aid your revision, not to replace it. The answers and explanations should not only provide a quick and concise revision aid but also work to develop your examination technique. Remember that it is very important to read the question thoroughly to avoid getting caught out!

Each mock paper is designed to be completed in 45 minutes. We hope you will find sitting each mock paper to time a useful form of self-assessment, reinforcing your revision. While the time-to-question ratio reflects that in the MRCS examination papers, we feel 45 minutes can be fitted into a busy revision schedule, between working long hours and having a bit of fun!

We hope you will enjoy this book and wish you patience with your revision and the best of luck in your future surgical careers!

Charlotte Dunford
Sarah Waldman
Zoe Barber
March 2013

About the authors

Charlotte Dunford MBBS BSc (Hons) MRCS
Charlotte's undergraduate medical training was at Imperial College, London. She completed her foundation training in the North West Thames Deanery and is currently a core surgical trainee in the Oxford Deanery.

Sarah Waldman MA (Cantab) MBBChir MRCS
Sarah's undergraduate medical training was at Cambridge University. She completed her foundation training in the Wessex Deanery and is currently an academic clinical fellow in general surgery in the Oxford Deanery.

Zoe Barber MA (Oxon) BM BCh MRCS
Zoe's undergraduate medical training was at Oxford University. She completed her foundation training and is currently a core surgical trainee in the Oxford Deanery.

Abbreviations

2,3-DPG	2,3-diphosphoglycerate
A&E	accident and emergency
ABG	arterial blood gas
ABPI	ankle brachial pressure index
ADH	antidiuretic hormone
AF	atrial fibrillation
ALT	alanine transaminase
AMTS	abbreviated mental test score
AP	antero-posterior
ATLS	Advanced Trauma Life Support
BE	base excess
BMI	body mass index
BP	blood pressure
BPAP	bi-level positive airway pressure
CA	cancer antigen
CEA	carcinoembryonic antigen
CNS	central nervous system
COPD	chronic obstructive pulmonary disease
COX	cyclo-oxygenase
CPAP	continuous positive airway pressure
CPP	cerebral perfusion pressure
CRP	C-reactive protein
CT	computed tomography
CVP	central venous pressure
DCIS	ductal carcinoma in situ
DIP	distal interphalangeal
DJ	duodenojejunal
DPL	diagnostic peritoneal lavage
DSA	digital subtraction angiography

ECG	electrocardiogram
ED	emergency department
FAP	familial adenomatous polyposis
FEV_1	forced expiratory volume in 1 second
FNA	fine-needle aspiration
FVC	forced vital capacity
GCS	Glasgow Coma Scale
GI	gastrointestinal
HNPCC	hereditary non-polyposis colorectal cancer
HR	heart rate
ICP	intracranial pressure
IL	interleukin
ICU	intensive care unit
IV	intravenous
LMWH	low-molecular-weight heparin
MAP	mean arterial pressure
MEN 1/2	multiple endocrine neoplasia type 1/2
MRA	magnetic resonance angiography
MRI	magnetic resonance imaging
NF	neurofibromatosis
NF1/2	neurofibromatosis type 1/2
NG	nasogastric
NICE	National Institute for Health and Clinical Excellence
NJ	nasojejunal
NSAIDs	non-steroidal anti-inflammatory drugs
$PaCO_2$	partial pressure of carbon dioxide
PCA	patient-controlled analgesia
PEFR	peak expiratory flow rate
PEG	percutaneous endoscopic gastrostomy
PGE2	prostaglandin E2
PIP	proximal interphalangeal
PLAP	placental alkaline phosphatase
pO_2	partial pressure of oxygen
PSA	prostate-specific antigen

PTH	parathyroid hormone
RR	respiratory rate
SIADH	syndrome of inappropriate antidiuretic hormone secretion
SIRS	systemic inflammatory response syndrome
TB	tuberculosis
TGF	transforming growth factor
TIA	transient ischaemic attack
TNF-alpha	tumour necrosis factor-alpha
TPN	total parenteral nutrition
TSH	thyroid-stimulating hormone
TUR	trans-urethral resection
UC	ulcerative colitis
USS	ultrasound scan
UTI	urinary tract infection
VAC	vacuum-assisted closure
VTE	venous thromboembolism
WCC	white cell count

MRCS Part A Paper 1

Mock Paper 1

Please select the single best answer from the five possible answers for each question.

Please answer all questions.

You have **45 minutes** to complete this paper.

1. Which of the following is derived from the first branchial (pharyngeal) arch?

   a. Hyoid bone

   b. Masseter muscle

   c. Posterior third of the tongue

   d. Posterior belly of digastric muscle

   e. Sternohyoid muscle

2. Which of the following is contained within the middle mediastinum?

   a. Left main bronchus

   b. Right main bronchus

   c. Pericardium

   d. Superior vena cava

   e. All of the above

3. A 65-year-old gentleman is referred to the vascular clinic with right buttock claudication after walking 40 m. He has no other symptoms. Angiography is requested. Given this clinical information, which vessel is most likely affected?

    a. Right common iliac artery

    b. Right internal iliac artery

    c. Right external iliac artery

    d. Right common femoral artery

    e. Right profunda femoris (deep femoral) artery

4. Which of the following is *not* a recognised risk factor for venous thromboembolism (VTE)?

    a. Malignancy

    b. Varicose veins

    c. Polytrauma

    d. Pregnancy

    e. Previous deep vein thrombosis

5. Which of the following is the most common form of thyroid cancer?

    a. Follicular carcinoma

    b. Medullary carcinoma

    c. Anaplastic carcinoma

    d. Papillary carcinoma

    e. Thyroid lymphoma

6. Following a right inguinal hernia repair, a male presents to clinic complaining of numbness over his right anterior scrotum and medial thigh. Which nerve is most likely to have been affected?

    a. Internal pudendal

    b. Ilioinguinal

    c. Iliohypogastric

    d. Genitofemoral

    e. Obturator

7. Which of the following arteries does *not* supply the breast?

    a. Lateral thoracic branch of axillary artery

    b. Thoracoacromial branch of axillary artery

    c. Intercostal arteries

    d. Superior epigastric artery

    e. Internal thoracic artery

8. Which of the following aortic branches is correctly paired with the corresponding vertebral level(s) at which it leaves the aorta?

    a. Gonadal arteries – L4

    b. Superior mesenteric artery – L2

    c. Inferior mesenteric artery – L4

    d. Inferior phrenic arteries – T11

    e. Coeliac trunk – T12/L1

9. Which of the following is *not* generally an indication for renal replacement therapy?

   a. Urea >30 mmol/L

   b. Hyperkalaemia >6 mmol/L

   c. Encephalopathy

   d. Sodium <130 mmol/L

   e. Fluid overload

10. A 25-year-old male is diagnosed with ureteric colic. Which of the
    following may *inhibit* the formation of renal calculi?

    a. Hypercalciuria

    b. Hypercitraturia

    c. *Pseudomonas* infection

    d. Hyperoxaluria

    e. Hyperuricuria

11. A 28-year-old male falls awkwardly while playing rugby and presents
    complaining of pain in his shoulder. His arm is adducted and inter-
    nally rotated and he has a visible depression over the shoulder joint.
    What injury is he most likely to have sustained?

    a. Posterior dislocation of the shoulder

    b. Acromioclavicular joint subluxation

    c. Anterior dislocation of the shoulder

    d. Fracture of surgical neck of the humerus

    e. Fracture of anatomical neck of the humerus

12. A 30-year-old male presents to the emergency department (ED) with a thunderclap headache. You suspect a subarachnoid haemorrhage. A computed tomography (CT) scan is performed and, as no abnormality is seen, you proceed to a lumbar puncture. Which bony landmarks do you use to identify the correct spinal level for your needle?

a. Iliac crests

b. Natal cleft and posterior costal margin

c. Sacrum and spinous processes

d. Posterior superior iliac spine

e. Ischial tuberosities

13. You are called to see a 65-year-old female nine days after her total hip replacement. She has been slow to mobilise. She appears acutely confused and drowsy. Recorded observations report a heart rate (HR) of 100 bpm, blood pressure (BP) of 135/73 mmHg, O_2 saturation of 92% on room air, respiratory rate (RR) of 20 breaths/min and temperature of 37.2°C. What is the most likely cause of her acute confusion?

a. Pulmonary embolus

b. Myocardial infarction

c. Cerebrovascular accident

d. Sepsis

e. Opiate overdose

14. An 80-year-old male undergoes an elective total hip replacement. He has an epidural and regular paracetamol prescribed for pain control. You are called to the ward 8 hours after his operation, as his BP is 70/40 mmHg and his HR is 50 bpm. His RR is normal, as are his O_2 saturations. His urine output has dropped from 50 to 15 mL/h. What is the most likely cause for this physiological insult?

   a. Post-operative haemorrhage

   b. Epidural

   c. Intra-operative volume loss

   d. Systemic inflammatory response syndrome (SIRS)

   e. Sepsis

15. A 19-year-old male injures his right leg in a road traffic accident, developing nerve damage. On average, how long would a peripheral nerve neurapraxia take to recover?

   a. 5–6 days

   b. 2–4 weeks

   c. 6–8 weeks

   d. 8–12 months

   e. >12 months

16. Which of the following bone tumours is associated with retinoblastoma syndrome?

   a. Osteoma

   b. Osteoid osteoma

   c. Osteoblastoma

   d. Ewing's sarcoma

   e. Osteosarcoma

17. Which of the following is the most common cause of aortic stenosis in the United Kingdom?

    a. Congenital bicuspid valve

    b. Marfan's syndrome

    c. Rheumatic fever

    d. Age-related sclerosis

    e. Infective endocarditis

18. Which of the following is true regarding tuberculosis (TB)?

    a. Haematoxylin and eosin staining is the staining test of choice for identifying the organism responsible.

    b. It may be transmitted from mother to child via breast milk.

    c. Non-caseating granulomata are characteristic of pulmonary TB.

    d. Tumour necrosis factor (TNF)-alpha is important for granuloma wall integrity.

    e. The lung is the only site of primary TB.

19. Which law describes the relationship between end-diastolic volume and stroke volume?

    a. Laplace's law

    b. Frank–Starling law

    c. Poiseuille's law

    d. Fick's law

    e. Courvoisier's law

20. Which of the following bone disorders is characterised by an isolated decrease in bone mineralisation?

    a. Osteomalacia

    b. Osteopenia

    c. Osteoporosis

    d. Paget's disease

    e. Osteopetrosis

21. A 40-year-old female presents with symptomatic hypercalcaemia. Blood tests reveal an elevated serum parathyroid hormone (PTH) level and elevated serum calcium. Which of the following pathologies is most likely to cause this biochemical abnormality?

    a. Chronic renal failure

    b. Malabsorption

    c. Osteomalacia

    d. Pregnancy

    e. Parathyroid adenoma

22. Which of the following hormones is secreted by the posterior pituitary?

    a. Oxytocin

    b. Adrenocorticotrophic hormone

    c. Thyroid-stimulating hormone (TSH)

    d. Growth hormone

    e. Prolactin

23. Which of the following relationships between biochemical mediator and clinical sign is true for acute inflammation?

    a. Complement – rubor (redness)

    b. Leukotrienes – calor (warmth)

    c. Prostaglandins – functio laesa (function loss)

    d. Nitric oxide – tumour (swelling)

    e. Prostaglandin E2 (PGE2) – dolor (pain)

24. Which of the following is a recognised cause of pancreatitis?

    a. Metoclopramide

    b. Ramipril

    c. Aspirin

    d. Paracetamol

    e. Budesonide

25. Which of the following statements is true regarding the cell cycle?

    a. DNA synthesis occurs in M phase.

    b. Chromosome replication occurs in S phase.

    c. Cell division starts in G_1 and continues to G_2 phase.

    d. Cells are quiescent in G_1 and G_2 phases.

    e. It comprises ten discrete phases.

26. Which of the following syndromes is correctly paired with the gene responsible for it?

    a. Multiple endocrine neoplasia type 2 (MEN 2) – MET gene

    b. Retinoblastoma – RET gene

    c. Li–Fraumeni – p53 gene

    d. Prostate cancer – NF1 gene

    e. Hereditary non-polyposis colorectal cancer (HNPCC) – APC gene

27. What structure passes through the foramen spinosum?

    a. Facial nerve

    b. Vagus nerve

    c. Internal carotid artery

    d. Middle meningeal artery

    e. Internal jugular vein

28. Which division of the trigeminal nerve supplies the temporal skin?

    a. Maxillary

    b. Ophthalmic

    c. Temporal

    d. Mandibular

    e. Zygomatic

29. When standing, the manubriosternal angle is the surface marker for which anatomical structure?

    a. Arch of aorta

    b. Left venous angle

    c. Division of right main bronchus

    d. Right recurrent laryngeal nerve

    e. First intercostal space

30. Regarding the brachial plexus, which of the following statements is true?

    a. The axillary nerve is a branch of the lateral cord.

    b. The median nerve is derived from branches of the medial and lateral cords.

    c. The long thoracic nerve is normally derived from spinal roots C6, 7 and 8.

    d. The medial, lateral and posterior cords are so-called from their relation to the subclavian artery.

    e. The medial cutaneous nerve of the forearm is a branch of the musculocutaneous nerve.

31. A 35-year-old female is taken for an emergency laparotomy following blunt force trauma. Which of the following structures is intra-peritoneal?

    a. Third part of the duodenum

    b. Ovaries

    c. Adrenal glands

    d. Head of pancreas

    e. Bladder

32. A 70-year-old female undergoes an elective left total knee replacement. Which structure, vulnerable during this operation, is the deepest in the popliteal fossa?

    a. Popliteal vein

    b. Tibial nerve

    c. Common peroneal nerve

    d. Popliteal artery

    e. Short saphenous vein

33. A 65-year-old male is admitted electively for an inguinal hernia repair. He has smoked for 30 years and asks you what effect this will have on him during his surgery. Which of the following statements is true regarding the effects of smoking?

    a. Microangiopathic changes result in impaired wound healing.

    b. The carboxyhaemoglobin present in smoke causes a right shift in the O_2–haemoglobin dissociation curve.

    c. Smoking reduces the HR and increases O_2 demand.

    d. Smoking boosts the immune system.

    e. Stopping smoking 24 hours before surgery has no effect on cardiovascular function.

34. A 25-year-old female undergoes a diagnostic laparoscopy procedure for persisting right iliac fossa pain. Which of the following statements regarding diathermy is true?

    a. The coagulation mode uses short bursts of high-voltage energy to desiccate tissue.

    b. Capacitance coupling requires direct contact with tissues.

    c. Patients should ideally be in contact with a grounded metal object.

    d. The presence of a pacemaker is an absolute contraindication to monopolar diathermy.

    e. Hybrid laparoscopic ports reduce the risk of capacitance coupling.

35. Following a sub-total colectomy for ulcerative colitis (UC), a patient is returned to the ward with an epidural. Which of the following statements is true?

a. Epidurals contain only local anaesthetics.

b. The epidural could cause post-operative hypotension.

c. Epidurals should provide complete sensory and motor blockade.

d. Bupivacaine acts on the enzyme cyclo-oxygenase (COX) to induce anaesthesia.

e. Patients with asthma should avoid having an epidural.

36. A 25-year-old female presents with a wound infection post appendicectomy. She is allergic to penicillin, in that it causes anaphylaxis. Which other antibiotic group should you consider avoiding?

a. Quinolones

b. Aminoglycosides

c. Macrolides

d. Cephalosporins

e. Tetracyclines

37. In the critically ill surgical patient, nutritional support should be considered when a patient has had insufficient dietary intake for 3 days or more. Which of the following statements is true?

a. The parenteral route is the preferred method of giving nutritional support.

b. The enteral route is always safe to use and is the most cost-effective route for administering nutritional support.

c. Percutaneous jejunostomy is a procedure to allow parenteral nutrition to be administered.

d. Aspiration is a common complication of enteral feeding.

e. Marked interstitial fluid loss is a commonly seen metabolic response to SIRS and sepsis.

38. A patient with gastric outlet obstruction and persistent vomiting has a metabolic alkalosis. This causes poor tissue oxygenation. What is the main mechanism behind this poor oxygenation?

   a. In response to the metabolic alkalosis, hypoventilation reduces partial pressure of CO_2 ($PaCO_2$) and, consequently, partial pressure of O_2 (pO_2) in the blood.

   b. Protons and chloride are lost in vomitus.

   c. Volume depletion due to excessive vomiting reduces haemoglobin concentration.

   d. Alkalosis shifts the O_2–haemoglobin dissociation curve to the left.

   e. There is increased bicarbonate absorption.

39. A 35-year-old male with a bimalleolar fracture of his ankle is immobilised in a backslab plaster. He is complaining of severe pain in his leg, despite the fact that you have split the cast down to the skin. At what compartment pressures would you consider performing a fasciotomy?

   a. >30 mmHg

   b. >40 mmHg

   c. >50 mmHg

   d. >60 mmHg

   e. >70 mmHg

40. What is the basic water requirement of an adult in good health?

   a. 10–20 mL/kg/day

   b. 20–30 mL/kg/day

   c. 30–40 mL/kg/day

   d. 40–50 mL/kg/day

   e. 50–60 mL/kg/day

41. A 65-year-old female with chronic obstructive pulmonary disease (COPD) requires an emergency laparotomy for ischaemic bowel. She develops an infective exacerbation of her COPD post-operatively. Her blood gas on air is as follows: pH 7.32; pO_2, 6.9; $PaCO_2$, 8.7; base excess (BE), −3.5; and HCO_3, 23. What type of respiratory support would be most appropriate?

    a. High-flow O_2 via a non-re-breather mask

    b. Continuous positive airway pressure (CPAP)

    c. Bi-level positive airway pressure (BPAP)

    d. Intubation and ventilation

    e. None of the above

42. Which of the following is a recognised risk factor for gastric cancer?

    a. Smoking

    b. Affected second-degree relative

    c. Female sex

    d. Barrett's oesophagus

    e. Blood type AB

43. An 18-year-old female presents with a lump in her right breast that she noticed while showering. She is otherwise well and takes no regular medication. The lump is 2 cm in diameter, smooth and firm. It is mobile. What is the most likely diagnosis?

    a. Fibroadenoma

    b. Fibrocystic change

    c. Ductal carcinoma in situ (DCIS)

    d. Carcinoma

    e. Fat necrosis

44. A 25-year-old type 1 diabetic male presents unwell, with a blood glucose measurement of 26 mmol/L. Examination reveals a HR of 110 bpm, BP of 110/60 mmHg and RR of 30 breaths/min. He appears severely dehydrated. What is the most likely acid–base abnormality you will find on arterial blood gas (ABG) sampling?

a. Metabolic alkalosis

b. Metabolic acidosis

c. Mixed metabolic and respiratory acidosis

d. Metabolic alkalosis with respiratory compensation

e. Metabolic acidosis with respiratory compensation

45. Which of the following shifts the O_2–haemoglobin dissociation curve to the left?

a. Decreased temperature

b. Decreased CO_2

c. The Haldane effect

d. Increased pH

e. All of the above

46. How long should be waited after a child is fed breast milk before administering general anaesthesia for an elective procedure?

a. 1 hour

b. 2 hours

c. 3 hours

d. 4 hours

e. 6 hours

47. A 25-year-old male pedestrian hit by a car is brought into the accident and emergency (A&E) department unconscious. He is making incomprehensible sounds and his eyes open in response to pain only. His right arm localises to a painful stimulus while his left arm only extends in response. What is his Glasgow Coma Scale (GCS) score?

    a. 6

    b. 7

    c. 8

    d. 9

    e. 10

48. Which of the following is an *absolute* contraindication to diagnostic peritoneal lavage (DPL)?

    a. Evisceration of bowel

    b. Morbid obesity

    c. Diagnostic uncertainty

    d. Previous laparotomy

    e. Pregnancy

49. A 50 kg 34-year-old female sustains third-degree burns to 40% of her body surface area. What should her intravenous (IV) fluid replacement for the first 8 hours be?

    a. 1600 mL

    b. 2000 mL

    c. 4000 mL

    d. 6600 mL

    e. 8000 mL

50. A patient complains of altered vision following an ischaemic stroke. On examination, you find a visual field defect affecting the left half of the visual field in both eyes. Where is the lesion?

    a. Right optic nerve

    b. Optic chiasm

    c. Left optic nerve

    d. Left optic tract

    e. Right optic tract

MRCS Part A Paper 1

Mock Paper 2

Please select the single best answer from the five possible answers for each question.

Please answer all questions.

You have **45 minutes** to complete this paper.

1. Each of the following structures passes through the diaphragm at a certain vertebral level. Which of the following pairings is correct?

   a. T12 – inferior vena cava

   b. T12 – azygos vein

   c. T10 – right phrenic nerve

   d. T8 – oesophagus

   e. T10 – aorta

2. Which of the following tumours is typically associated with multiple endocrine neoplasia type 1 (MEN 1)?

   a. Prolactinoma

   b. Medullary thyroid carcinoma

   c. Phaeochromocytoma

   d. Mucocutaneous fibroma

   e. None of the above

3. A 70-year-old female undergoes emergency surgery for ischaemic bowel. A large section of ascending colon has to be resected. Which artery supplies this area of the bowel?

   a. Coeliac

   b. Inferior mesenteric

   c. Lower left colic

   d. Superior mesenteric

   e. Superior epigastric

4. Which of the following structures is part of the spermatic cord?

   a. Testicular artery

   b. Pampiniform plexus

   c. Sympathetic nerves

   d. Cremasteric artery

   e. All of the above

5. What is the most common cardiac abnormality seen on an electrocardiogram (ECG) in a patient with a pulmonary embolism?

   a. T wave inversion in any lead

   b. S wave in lead 1

   c. Q wave in lead 3

   d. Sinus tachycardia

   e. ST elevation in any lead

6. A 16-year-old female presents with chronic diarrhoea and abdominal pain. She is investigated for inflammatory bowel disease. Which of the following would be most likely to indicate a diagnosis of UC?

   a. Presence of significant jejunal inflammation

   b. Presence of non-caseating granulomata in the bowel wall

   c. Presence of multiple perianal fistulas

   d. Fatty encroachment of the serosal layer of the bowel wall

   e. Inflammation confined to the mucosal and submucosal layers of the bowel wall

7. A 30-year-old male has dislocated his shoulder playing football. He reports reduced sensation over the regimental patch on the affected side. Which nerve is most likely to have been affected?

   a. Axillary nerve

   b. Musculocutaneous nerve

   c. Lateral cutaneous nerve of the arm

   d. Lateral pectoral nerve

   e. Nerve to subclavius

8. You are called to see a 75-year-old male 5 hours after a transurethral resection (TUR) of the prostate. He is very drowsy and acutely confused when nurses try to wake him. He has a medical history of transient ischaemic attacks (TIAs). On examination, you find his RR is 8 breaths/min. What is the most likely cause of his symptoms?

   a. TUR of the prostate syndrome

   b. Opiate overdose

   c. Myocardial infarction

   d. Pulmonary embolus

   e. Hypoxia

9. The pathophysiological principle of wound healing by secondary intention involves which of the following?

   a. Tissue grafts

   b. Wound-edge approximation

   c. Sutures

   d. Granulation tissue formation

   e. Vacuum-assisted closure (VAC) dressing

10. Which of the following vasculitides is most likely to be associated with the development of an abdominal aortic aneurysm?

    a. Churg–Strauss syndrome

    b. Polyarteritis nodosa

    c. Takayasu's arteritis

    d. Henoch–Schönlein purpura

    e. Wegener's granulomatosis

11. Which of the following conditions causes clotting dysfunction via factor IX deficiency?

    a. Haemophilia A

    b. Von Willebrand's disease

    c. Glanzmann's disease

    d. Haemophilia B

    e. Bernard–Soulier syndrome

12. Which of the following is true regarding neurofibromatosis (NF)?

    a. Inheritance is autosomal recessive.

    b. Acoustic neuromas are seen in neurofibromatosis type 2 (NF2).

    c. There are only two forms of NF.

    d. Schwannomas are seen in neurofibromatosis type 1 (NF1).

    e. Café au lait spots are seen in NF2.

13. Which of the following is typically associated with osteoarthritis?

    a. Pannus

    b. Bouchard's nodes

    c. Swan neck deformity

    d. Boutonniere's deformity

    e. Tophi

14. Which of the following conditions is typically associated with a transudative pleural effusion?

    a. Pneumonia

    b. Rheumatoid arthritis

    c. Meigs' syndrome

    d. Pancreatitis

    e. Pulmonary embolism

15. Which of the following is an example of non-cyanotic congenital heart disease?

    a. Eisenmenger's syndrome

    b. Tetralogy of Fallot

    c. Persistent truncus arteriosus

    d. Ventricular septal defect

    e. Hypoplastic left heart syndrome

16. Which part of the heart has the fastest intrinsic firing rate?

    a. Atrium

    b. Purkinje fibres

    c. Atrioventricular node

    d. Bundle of His

    e. Sino-atrial node

17. A patient is noted to be hypertensive and undergoes blood tests. They reveal raised serum sodium and low serum potassium levels. Plasma renin levels are reduced. What is the most likely cause of this?

    a. Heart failure

    b. Liver cirrhosis

    c. Nephrotic syndrome

    d. Adrenal cortical adenoma

    e. Phaeochromocytoma

18. Regarding the shoulder joint, which of the following rotator cuff insertions is correct?

    a. The supraspinatus inserts onto the most superior part of the lesser tubercle of the humerus.

    b. The subscapularis inserts onto the most inferior part of the greater tubercle of the humerus.

    c. The teres minor inserts onto the most inferior part of the greater tubercle of the humerus.

    d. The infraspinatus inserts onto the most superior part of the greater tubercle of the humerus.

    e. None of the above.

19. Which of the following is true regarding the microscopic appearances of acute inflammation?

    a. C5a is chemotactic.

    b. Macrophages are the predominant cell type in the first 24 hours.

    c. Smooth muscle relaxation is predominantly due to histamine release.

    d. C3b increases vascular permeability.

    e. Formation of the membrane attack complex is initiated by nitric oxide.

20. At which stage of mitosis does chromosome replication result in 96 chromosomes in each cell?

    a. Interphase

    b. Prophase

    c. Metaphase

    d. Anaphase

    e. Telophase

21. Which of the following tumour markers is correctly paired with its specific cancer?

    a. Cancer antigen (CA) 125 – breast cancer

    b. CA 15-3 – ovarian cancer

    c. CA 19-9 – choriocarcinoma

    d. Carcinoembryonic antigen (CEA) – sarcoma

    e. Placental alkaline phosphatase (PLAP) – seminoma

22. Which of the following statements regarding statistical data is true?

    a. The mean is a measure of data spread.

    b. The mode is a measure of data location.

    c. The median is the most commonly occurring value in a data set.

    d. A median can be used with nominal data.

    e. A mean cannot be used with ordinal data.

23. Which of the following structures travels through the sphenoid bone?

    a. Maxillary branch of trigeminal nerve

    b. Internal carotid artery

    c. Optic nerve

    d. Vestibulocochlear nerve

    e. Facial nerve

24. What structure passes into the foramen lacerum?

    a. Internal jugular vein

    b. Glossopharyngeal nerve

    c. Vagus nerve

    d. Internal carotid artery

    e. Middle meningeal artery

25. A patient complains of double vision when looking to the right. On examination, you find he cannot abduct his right eye. A CT scan of the head reveals an aneurysm of the intercavernous internal carotid artery. Which nerve is most likely to be affected?

    a. Abducens

    b. Oculomotor

    c. Trochlear

    d. Nasociliary

    e. Optic

26. Following excision of the right salivary gland post infection, a patient complains of asymmetry in their smile and weakness in the lower lip. Which nerve is affected?

    a. Maxillary branch of the trigeminal nerve

    b. Nerve to mylohyoid

    c. Lingual nerve

    d. Marginal mandibular branch of the facial nerve

    e. Hypoglossal nerve

27. You are called to see a patient who is unwell post-operatively. As part of your assessment, you auscultate the chest. Which of the following is most likely to be true?

a. The aortic valve is auscultated in the left second intercostal space.

b. The mitral valve is auscultated in the left parasternal area, fourth intercostal space.

c. The middle lobe of the right lung is best auscultated in the right axilla.

d. The inferior lobe of the left lung is best auscultated posteriorly.

e. The horizontal fissure of the left lung extends from the oblique fissure in the fourth intercostal space to the anterior costal cartilage.

28. A 53-year-old female undergoes a mastectomy and axillary node clearance. Which of the following statements is true?

a. Damage to the thoracodorsal nerve causes winging of the scapula.

b. Axillary lymph nodes are divided into levels according to their relationship to pectoralis major.

c. The surface marking of the breast extends from the parasternal line to the anterior axillary line.

d. The majority of breast lymphatic drainage is to the parasternal lymph nodes.

e. Sensation to the breast and nipple is from the 4th to the 6th intercostal nerve.

29. A 28-year-old male with Crohn's disease has developed a small bowel obstruction. Investigations suggest there is a transition point in the proximal bowel at the jejunoileal junction. Intra-operatively, how can you distinguish the jejunum from the ileum?

    a. The ileum is darker in colour than the jejunum.

    b. Lumen size increases distally from jejunum to ileum.

    c. The jejunum is more vascular than the ileum.

    d. The ileum has much longer vasa recta than the jejunum.

    e. The jejunum has more fat in the mesentery than the ileum.

30. A 55-year-old male admitted with acute pancreatitis has a CT scan and is found to have developed a pseudocyst. Incidentally, the CT scan also shows that the patient has nephrocalcinosis. Which blood test should you order to determine whether the two conditions have the same underlying aetiology?

    a. Serum potassium

    b. Serum amylase

    c. Serum urate

    d. Serum calcium

    e. Serum phosphate

31. A 20-year-old motorcyclist involved in a road traffic accident suffers a mid-shaft femoral fracture. How many fascial compartments are there in the thigh?

    a. Two

    b. Three

    c. Four

    d. Five

    e. Six

32. A 45-year-old male presents with difficulty in walking. On examination, he is found to have a Trendelenburg gait. Which nerve is most likely to be affected?

    a. Obturator

    b. Superior gluteal

    c. Sciatic

    d. Inferior gluteal

    e. Femoral

33. A 70-year-old male is admitted following an acute myocardial infarction requiring thrombolysis. He is due to have an elective total hip replacement in 2 weeks, but this is cancelled. What is the most likely reason for the cancellation of the surgery?

    a. His reduced exercise tolerance will impair post-operative mobilisation.

    b. There is an increased risk of intra-operative blood loss.

    c. Monopolar diathermy is absolutely contraindicated.

    d. There is a ~75% risk of further myocardial infarction intra-operatively.

    e. Intubation will be technically very difficult.

34. A 45-year-old type 1 diabetic who also has chronic kidney disease stage III presents with renal colic. She has a positive urine dipstick for nitrites, leucocytes, protein and blood. She is allergic to co-trimoxazole. Which antibiotic should be considered for treatment in this case?

    a. Linezolid

    b. Amoxicillin/clavulanic acid

    c. Trimethoprim

    d. Nitrofurantoin

    e. Vancomycin

35. A 60-year-old male is in septic shock with a perforated gallbladder. Which of the following parameters defines 'cardiovascular system failure' or 'dysfunction'?

   a. Urine output <120 mL over 4 hours

   b. Confusion with a GCS score <15

   c. Hypoxia with pO_2 <9.3 kPa

   d. Pyrexia with a temperature >38°C

   e. Lactate >12 mmol/L

36. A 35-year-old female with Crohn's disease presents with a small bowel obstruction. She has had multiple resections and has approximately 200 cm of small bowel left. She has a body mass index (BMI) of 18 and has not eaten properly for the last week. What would be the most appropriate route through which to start feeding?

   a. Nasogastric (NG) tube

   b. Percutaneous endoscopic jejunostomy (PEJ)

   c. Percutaneous endoscopic gastrostomy (PEG)

   d. Central line

   e. Oral

37. What is the minimum urine output that should be achieved by a normal adult?

   a. 0.2 mL/kg/h

   b. 0.5 mL/kg/h

   c. 1.0 mL/kg/h

   d. 1.5 mL/kg/h

   e. 2.0 mL/kg/h

38. Which of the following may cause hypernatraemia?

    a. Conn's syndrome

    b. Cushing's syndrome

    c. Diabetes insipidus

    d. Dehydration

    e. All of the above

39. Which of the following is a hormone involved in calcium metabolism that is produced by parafollicular C cells?

    a. Calcitonin

    b. Vitamin D

    c. 1,25-dihydroxycholecalciferol

    d. Parathormone-related peptide

    e. Parathyroid hormone

40. A 74-year-old female has noted scaly, itchy skin involving her left nipple. She is otherwise well and takes no regular medication. There is no discharge, no underlying lump and no lymphadenopathy. The nipple itself is red and scaly. The right nipple appears unaffected. What is the most likely diagnosis?

    a. Eczema

    b. Duct ectasia

    c. Fibrocystic change

    d. Paget's disease of the nipple

    e. Cellulitis

41. Which of the following shifts the O_2–haemoglobin dissociation curve to the left?

    a. Increased pH

    b. Increased CO_2

    c. Increased temperature

    d. Reduced tissue perfusion

    e. Increased 2,3-diphosphoglycerate (2,3-DPG)

42. An 18-year-old female presents following a deliberate overdose of aspirin. She is unsure how many tablets she has taken. Her HR is 95 bpm, BP is 125/70 mmHg and RR is 30 breaths/min. What acid–base abnormality are you most likely to find on initial ABG sampling?

    a. Metabolic alkalosis

    b. Metabolic acidosis

    c. Respiratory alkalosis

    d. Respiratory acidosis

    e. Mixed respiratory and metabolic alkalosis

43. A 40-year-old female presents with a femoral hernia. What is the lateral border of the femoral canal?

    a. Femoral nerve

    b. Lacunar ligament

    c. Inguinal ligament

    d. Femoral vein

    e. Femoral artery

44. A patient's blood tests show that they have a raised serum CA 125. This tumour marker is sometimes associated with cancer of which organ?

    a. Bowel

    b. Breast

    c. Pancreas

    d. Stomach

    e. Ovary

45. Which of the following statements is true regarding ulcerative colitis (UC)?

    a. It is common to see skip lesions in UC patients.

    b. Smoking is a positive risk factor for the development of UC.

    c. It affects the full thickness of the bowel wall.

    d. It is a risk factor for the development of bowel cancer.

    e. It is characterised by the presence of non-caseating granulomata.

46. A patient attends clinic with a suspected inguinal hernia. What is the surface marking of the deep inguinal ring?

    a. Halfway between the pubic symphysis and the greater trochanter of the femur

    b. Above and medial to the pubic tubercle

    c. Below and lateral to the pubic tubercle

    d. Halfway between the pubic tubercle and the anterior superior iliac spine

    e. The mid-inguinal point

47. Which of the following is a risk factor for developmental dysplasia of the hip?

a. Male sex

b. Polyhydramnios

c. Firstborn child

d. Cephalic presentation

e. African origin

48. A patient with an epidural complains of abdominal pain following a caesarean section. You test the sensory level and find it to be at the level of the umbilicus. What dermatome is this most likely to be?

a. T6

b. T8

c. T10

d. T12

e. L2

49. A 26-year-old female with familial adenomatous polyposis (FAP) attends clinic. She is concerned about the risk of passing FAP on to her children. Her mother also had FAP but her father was unaffected. What is the risk of her first child developing the disease, assuming the father is not affected?

a. 0.0%

b. 12.5%

c. 25.0%

d. 50.0%

e. 75.0%

50. Which of the following is the least common thyroid cancer in the United Kingdom?

a. Follicular carcinoma

b. Papillary carcinoma

c. Lymphoma

d. Medullary carcinoma

e. Anaplastic carcinoma

MRCS Part A Paper 1

Mock Paper 3

Please select the single best answer from the five possible answers for each question.

Please answer all questions.

You have **45 minutes** to complete this paper.

1. Which of the following structures is *least* likely to be damaged during an open total thyroidectomy?

    a. Recurrent laryngeal nerve

    b. Parathyroid gland

    c. Superior laryngeal nerve

    d. Superior thyroid artery

    e. External carotid artery

2. Which of the following shifts the O_2–haemoglobin dissociation curve to the right?

    a. Decreased temperature

    b. Decreased CO_2

    c. Haldane effect

    d. Increased 2,3-DPG

    e. All of the above

3. Which of the following is a form of primary lung cancer?

    a. Adenocarcinoma

    b. Bronchoalveolar carcinoma

    c. Carcinoid

    d. Oat cell carcinoma

    e. All of the above

4. A 24-year-old with a testicular tumour undergoes staging investigations. Which lymph nodes do the testes drain to?

    a. Inguinal

    b. Iliac

    c. Para-aortic

    d. Femoral

    e. Inferior mesenteric

5. A 58-year-old female is admitted following an upper gastrointestinal (GI) bleed. An oesophagogastroduodenoscopy is performed and she is found to have a peptic ulcer on the posterior wall of the first part of the duodenum. Which vessel is likely to be the source of the bleeding?

    a. Right gastric artery

    b. Gastroduodenal artery

    c. Left gastric vein

    d. Superior pancreaticoduodenal artery

    e. Superior mesenteric vein

6. Which three features of breast cancer provide the best indicator of prognosis?

   a. The size of the primary tumour, the grade of the tumour and the involvement of lymph nodes

   b. The size of the primary tumour, the oestrogen-receptor status and the grade of the tumour

   c. The grade of the tumour, the involvement of lymph nodes and the degree of vascular invasion

   d. The grade of the tumour, the degree of vascular invasion and the oestrogen-receptor status

   e. The size of the primary tumour, the involvement of lymph nodes and the degree of vascular invasion

7. Following a routine long saphenous vein ligation and stripping, a patient complains of numbness over the inner aspect of his ankle. Which nerve is most likely to have been affected?

   a. Sural

   b. Saphenous

   c. Anterior tibial

   d. Deep peroneal

   e. Obturator

8. A 66-year-old female is undergoing a left carpal tunnel decompression under local anaesthetic. You seek the patient's consent for the procedure, informing her that a risk is loss of sensation to the thenar eminence. Which nerve is most likely to be involved in this complication?

   a. Anterior interosseous nerve

   b. Recurrent branch of the median nerve

   c. Palmar cutaneous branch of the median nerve

   d. Lateral cutaneous nerve of the forearm

   e. Radial nerve

9. A 30-year-old male is brought into the ED following a head injury. As part of his initial resuscitation, he is intubated and ventilated. To prevent secondary brain injury, his $PaCO_2$ should ideally be kept at what level?

    a. 2.0–3.5 kPa

    b. 3.0–3.5 kPa

    c. 4.0–4.5 kPa

    d. 4.5–5.5 kPa

    e. 5.5–6.0 kPa

10. A 75-year-old male undergoes an elective total knee replacement. He has a 60-pack-year smoking history. Five days after his operation, he becomes confused and agitated. His BP drops to 80/40 mmHg, his HR is 110, he saturates at 90% on room air and his temperature is 38.5°C. What is the most likely cause of his symptoms?

    a. Urine infection

    b. Wound infection

    c. Chest infection

    d. Dehydration

    e. Atelectasis

11. Which of the following growth factors is *not* involved in wound healing and granulation tissue formation?

    a. Fibroblast growth factor

    b. Transforming growth factor (TGF)

    c. Platelet-derived growth factor

    d. Vascular endothelial growth factor

    e. Insulin-like growth factor

12. Which of the following is most likely to be associated with a mycotic aortic aneurysm?
    a. *Streptococcus viridans*
    b. *Staphylococcus aureus*
    c. *Streptococcus bovis*
    d. *Treponema pallidum*
    e. *Neisseria gonorrhoeae*

13. Which of the following may be a cause of communicating hydrocephalus?
    a. Choroid plexus tumour
    b. Arnold–Chiari malformation
    c. Atresia of the foramen of Magendie
    d. Congenital stenosis of the cerebral aqueduct
    e. Dandy–Walker malformation

14. Which of the following radiographic changes is most likely to be associated with rheumatoid arthritis?
    a. Subchondral sclerosis
    b. Subchondral cysts
    c. Joint subluxation
    d. Osteophytes
    e. Pathological fractures

15. Which of the following cardiac abnormalities forms part of the tetralogy of Fallot?
    a. Atrial septal defect
    b. Left ventricular hypertrophy
    c. Tricuspid atresia
    d. Overriding pulmonary artery
    e. Pulmonary stenosis

16. Which of the following endocrine disorders is most commonly associated with hypertension?

    a. Waterhouse–Friderichsen syndrome

    b. Addison's disease

    c. Sheehan's syndrome

    d. Conn's syndrome

    e. Diabetes insipidus

17. Which of the following disorders is characterised by the presence of thyroid peroxidase antibodies in serum?

    a. Graves' disease

    b. Hashimoto's thyroiditis

    c. De Quervain's thyroiditis

    d. Subacute lymphocytic thyroiditis

    e. Anaplastic carcinoma of the thyroid

18. A patient with hyponatraemia undergoes additional tests. Clinically, they are euvolaemic. Further testing reveals high urinary osmolality. Which of the following is the most likely cause of these biochemical abnormalities?

    a. Addison's disease

    b. Nephrotic syndrome

    c. Syndrome of inappropriate antidiuretic hormone secretion (SIADH)

    d. Frusemide use

    e. Thiazide diuretic use

19. Which of the following is true regarding nephroblastoma (Wilms' tumour)?

    a. It is commonly bilateral.

    b. It occurs more commonly in adults than children.

    c. It has a poor prognosis (<50% 5-year survival).

    d. It is the most common intra-abdominal tumour of childhood.

    e. Radiotherapy is the primary mode of therapy for stage 1 disease.

20. A patient presents with Wilson's disease, a copper metabolism disorder. Which protein is copper bound to in plasma?

    a. Albumin

    b. Caeruloplasmin

    c. Haptoglobin

    d. Apolipoprotein

    e. Transferrin

21. Which of these statements is correct regarding the pathology of chronic inflammation?

    a. Neutrophils are the predominant cell type.

    b. Interleukin (IL)-6 activates fibroblasts, resulting in scarring.

    c. TNF-alpha stimulates fibrosis.

    d. Natural killer T cells activate B lymphocytes to produce plasma cells.

    e. Plasma cells produce antibodies against the persistent antigen.

22. Which of the following statements regarding thyroid cancer is true?

    a. Follicular carcinoma can be diagnosed by fine-needle aspiration (FNA).

    b. Follicular carcinoma is the most common thyroid malignancy.

    c. Medullary carcinoma is derived from C cells.

    d. Papillary carcinoma commonly metastasises.

    e. Anaplastic carcinoma is associated with MEN 2 syndrome.

23. A toxin released from which of the following scorpions may cause acute pancreatitis?

    a. *Tityus tenuicauda*

    b. *Tityus trinitatis*

    c. *Tityus stigmurus*

    d. *Tityus serrulatus*

    e. *Tityus pintodarochai*

24. In mitosis, chromosomes move to opposite poles of the cell under the control of what structures?

    a. Histones

    b. Mitochondria

    c. Microtubules

    d. Golgi apparatuses

    e. Lysosomes

25. Which of the following statements regarding statistical data is true?

    a. Non-parametric tests analyse normally distributed data.

    b. 'Specificity' is the ability of a test to correctly identify those with a disease.

    c. If a study is adequately powered, this lessens the chance of obtaining a false-negative result.

    d. Type I errors occur when a test identifies a false negative.

    e. 'Confounding' identifies the strength of association between two variables.

26. Which of these structures passes through the foramen magnum?

    a. Spinal roots of the accessory nerve

    b. Facial nerve

    c. Mandibular division of the trigeminal nerve

    d. Internal carotid artery

    e. Internal jugular vein

27. Following an injury to the left side of the head, a patient complains of double vision, which is worse when descending stairs. The patient can compensate by tilting their head to the right. Which nerve is most likely to be affected?

    a. Oculomotor

    b. Trochlear

    c. Abducens

    d. Nasociliary

    e. Optic

28. Which nerve supplies the skin over the mastoid, pinna and angle of the jaw?

    a. Mandibular division of trigeminal

    b. Mandibular branch of facial

    c. Temporal

    d. Zygomatic

    e. Great auricular

29. You are called to the ward to see a patient post-operatively. The nurses are concerned that his RR is 28 breaths/min. Which of the following statements regarding the mechanics of breathing is true?

    a. Expiration is essentially a passive process involving relaxation of the diaphragm and elastic recoil of the lungs.

    b. Bucket-handle movement of the chest occurs mainly at the vertebra-sternal ribs.

    c. 'Pump handle' movement of the ribs increases the transverse dimension of the chest wall more than the antero-posterior dimension.

    d. The external intercostal muscles are the predominant muscles of respiration.

    e. Nerve supply to the intercostal muscles is derived from spinal roots C3–5.

30. A 45-year-old female with breast cancer undergoes chemotherapy. A Hickman line is inserted in the right subclavian vein. Which of the following statements is true?

a. The subclavian vein runs behind the subclavian artery.

b. There is a risk of damaging the thoracic duct on the right side.

c. On cannulation of the vein, the needle will pass through the sternal head of pectoralis major.

d. The subclavian vein and external jugular vein join to form the brachiocephalic vein.

e. The subclavian vein runs between the subclavius and anterior scalene muscles.

31. A 48-year-old female undergoes a wide local excision and axillary node sampling. Intra-operatively, large bulky lymph nodes are found and dissection is difficult. Post-operatively, she complains of weakness in the arm. On examination, you note she has weakness in adduction and internal rotation of the affected arm. Which nerve is most likely to be affected?

a. Thoracodorsal

b. Long thoracic

c. Medial pectoral

d. Axillary

e. Lateral pectoral

32. A patient is having an elective laparoscopic cholecystectomy. He is a type 1 diabetic and requires a sliding scale. You are asked to insert a cannula into the antecubital fossa. Which of the following statements is most likely to be true?

    a. The median cubital vein is present in all patients.

    b. The median nerve is situated medial to the brachial artery.

    c. The brachial artery is situated lateral to the biceps tendon.

    d. The floor of the cubital fossa is the brachioradialis.

    e. The pronator teres is situated laterally in the cubital fossa.

33. A 55-year-old female undergoes a cystectomy for carcinoma in situ. Which of the following structures can be damaged in this patient when the ureter is divided near its insertion into the bladder?

    a. Ilioinguinal nerve

    b. Genitofemoral nerve

    c. Dorsal venous complex

    d. Uterine artery

    e. External pudendal artery

34. What condition is most likely to ensue following damage to the middle meningeal artery?

    a. Venous sinus thrombosis

    b. Subdural haematoma

    c. Extradural haematoma

    d. Transient ischaemic attack

    e. Subarachnoid haemorrhage

35. An 85-year-old undergoes a laparoscopic right hemicolectomy. What measures should be taken in the operating theatre to reduce the risk of developing a deep vein thrombosis?

    a. Wrapping the arms across the chest

    b. Pneumatic compression devices on the legs

    c. Gel cushions on dependent areas

    d. Use of a Bair Hugger®

    e. Placing the arms by the patient's side

36. A 65-year-old male presents with urosepsis. Your local policy suggests treatment with an aminoglycoside. Which of the following is an example of an aminoglycoside?

    a. Erythromycin

    b. Vancomycin

    c. Teicoplanin

    d. Linezolid

    e. Amikacin

37. A 65-year-old female with an enterocutaneous fistula requires total parenteral nutrition (TPN). Vitamins are added to the TPN. Which of the following is an example of a water-soluble vitamin?

    a. Vitamin C

    b. Vitamin A

    c. Vitamin K

    d. Vitamin E

    e. Vitamin D

38. A fit and well 73-year-old female returns from theatre recovery after repair of a strangulated femoral hernia. Her urine output has been 30 mL in the last 2 hours. What is the most common reason for oliguria in the post-operative patient?

a. Renal tubular dysfunction

b. Poor renal perfusion due to under-filling

c. Physiological stress response

d. Blocked urinary catheter

e. Intra-abdominal hypertension

39. Which of the following is a risk factor for post-operative atelectasis?

a. Obesity

b. Poor mobility

c. Abdominal surgery

d. Poorly controlled pain

e. All of the above

40. A 63-year-old female presents with a hard, painful breast lump that she noticed after banging into a door at work. She is hypertensive, a smoker and perimenopausal. The lump is 3 × 4 cm, firm and regular. You presume it to be fat necrosis. What is the most appropriate next step?

a. Reassurance

b. Mammography

c. Ultrasound scan (USS) and FNA

d. Mammography and FNA

e. Incision and drainage

41. You are considering performing a laparoscopic cholecystectomy on a patient with cardiac failure. What effect does a pneumoperitoneum have on the circulatory system?

    a. Increases preload

    b. Decreases afterload

    c. Decreases preload

    d. Increases afterload

    e. Affects both preload and afterload

42. What is ibuprofen's mechanism of action?

    a. Non-selective COX inhibition

    b. Lipoxygenase inhibition

    c. COX-2 inhibition

    d. COX-1 inhibition

    e. Phospholipase A inhibition

43. A 38-year-old female attends clinic with varicose veins. You assess the competence of her sapheno-femoral junction with a Doppler probe. What are the surface markings of the sapheno-femoral junction?

    a. 5 cm below and lateral to the pubic tubercle

    b. 5 cm medial to the femoral pulse

    c. 2 cm below and lateral to the pubic tubercle

    d. 1 cm lateral to the femoral pulse

    e. Directly over the femoral pulse

44. A patient complains of diplopia when walking downstairs but has not noticed it at any other time. Which nerve is most likely to be affected?

a. Abducens nerve

b. Oculomotor nerve

c. Facial nerve

d. Trochlear nerve

e. Optic nerve

45. A patient who was admitted with bleeding per rectum is mistakenly given a large dose of unfractionated heparin. Which of the following acts as a reversal agent for heparin?

a. Fresh frozen plasma

b. Cryoprecipitate

c. Protamine

d. Vitamin K

e. All of the above

46. An 8-year-old female falls off her bicycle and sustains a supracondylar fracture to her right humerus. She has difficulty making a fist and complains of altered sensation across the thenar eminence. Which nerve is most likely to be damaged here?

a. Ulnar nerve

b. Median nerve

c. Radial nerve

d. Axillary nerve

e. Musculocutaneous nerve

47. A 25-year-old singer undergoes a thyroidectomy. After the operation she notices that she can no longer sing high notes. Which nerve has been affected?

   a. Recurrent laryngeal

   b. Glossopharyngeal

   c. External laryngeal

   d. Internal laryngeal

   e. Hypoglossal

48. A patient undergoes a laparotomy for a traumatic liver laceration. There is extensive bleeding that becomes difficult to control. To gain control, the surgeon compresses an artery running along the free edge of the lesser omentum. Which artery is this?

   a. Cystic

   b. Right gastroduodenal

   c. Common hepatic

   d. Right gastric

   e. Superior mesenteric

49. A 65-year-old male develops osteomyelitis following a traumatic injury to his leg. Which organism is most likely responsible?

   a. *Haemophilus influenzae*

   b. *Staphylococcus aureus*

   c. *Escherichia coli*

   d. *Streptococcus pyogenes*

   e. *Staphylococcus epidermidis*

50. A 30-year-old male sustains a proximal tibial fracture during a road traffic accident. Once able to mobilise, he walks with a high-stepping action and notices loss of sensation on the dorsal aspect of his foot and the lateral aspect of his lower leg. On examination, you find he is unable to dorsiflex the ankle or evert the foot, but inversion is intact. Which nerve has been affected?

a. Femoral

b. Deep peroneal

c. Common peroneal

d. Tibial

e. Superficial peroneal

MRCS Part A Paper 1

Mock Paper 4

Please select the single best answer from the five possible answers for each question.

Please answer all questions.

You have **45 minutes** to complete this paper.

1. Which of the following is a centrally acting antihypertensive?

    a. Amlodipine

    b. Furosemide

    c. Spironolactone

    d. Clonidine

    e. Diltiazem

2. Which of the following hormones is produced by the adrenal cortex?

    a. Aldosterone

    b. Corticosterone

    c. Cortisol

    d. Dehydroepiandrosterone

    e. All of the above

3. Which of the following thyroid cancers generally has the worst prognosis?

   a. Medullary carcinoma

   b. Follicular carcinoma

   c. Anaplastic carcinoma

   d. Follicular adenoma

   e. Papillary carcinoma

4. Which of the following organisms is most likely to cause infective endocarditis?

   a. *Haemophilus influenzae*

   b. *Streptococcus viridans*

   c. *Staphylococcus bovis*

   d. *Escherichia coli*

   e. *Klebsiella pneumoniae*

5. Which of the following is true regarding the epiploic foramen?

   a. The posterior border is formed by the peritoneum over the inferior vena cava.

   b. The free edge of the greater omentum forms the anterior border.

   c. The third part of the duodenum forms the inferior border.

   d. The quadrate lobe of the liver lies superiorly.

   e. The portal triad lies anteriorly, within the greater omentum.

6. In which order do the structures of the kidney hilum lie in, anterior to posterior?

   a. Renal vein, renal artery, ureter

   b. Renal vein, ureter, renal artery

   c. Ureter, renal vein, renal artery

   d. Ureter, renal artery, renal vein

   e. Renal artery, ureter, renal vein

7. Intrinsic factor is secreted from which cells?

   a. G cells in the stomach

   b. Parietal cells in the terminal ileum

   c. Enterochromaffin-like cells in the stomach

   d. Enterochromaffin-like cells in the terminal ileum

   e. Parietal cells in the stomach

8. Which of the following is *not* a known risk factor for breast cancer?

   a. Breastfeeding a child for more than 6 months

   b. Menarche before the age of 12 years old

   c. Taking the combined oral contraceptive pill

   d. Strong family history of breast cancer

   e. Personal history of breast cancer

9. Following a comminuted mid-shaft humeral fracture, an 80-year-old female complains her grip has weakened on the affected side. She is still able to abduct and adduct her fingers. Which nerve is most likely to have been affected?

   a. Ulnar

   b. Radial

   c. Median

   d. Anterior interosseous

   e. Recurrent branch of the median

10. Following an inguinal hernia repair, a 30-year-old male complains of pain over the outer aspect of his thigh on the affected side. Which nerve is most likely to have been affected?

    a. Obturator nerve

    b. Ilioinguinal nerve

    c. Iliohypogastric nerve

    d. Lateral cutaneous nerve of the thigh

    e. Inferior gluteal nerve

11. A 55-year-old male plays cricket and is a bowler for the local team. He presents with some difficulty in moving his shoulder. On examination, you find he initiates abduction by leaning his body out to the side. Which muscle is most likely affected?

    a. Deltoid

    b. Teres major

    c. Supraspinatus

    d. Teres minor

    e. Pectoralis major

12. A 30-year-old male is brought into the ED with a head injury. What is the best position for his bed to be in during the initial stages of his management?

    a. 30 degrees head down

    b. Supine

    c. 45 degrees head up

    d. 45 degrees head down

    e. 30 degrees head up

13. A 77-year-old male presents to the ED 5 days after a femoro-distal bypass in his right leg. The wound is red and indurated and the whole limb has swollen. The patient is pyrexial and tachycardic. He has not passed urine for the last 18 hours. There is no palpable bladder clinically. What would be your initial step in assessing the patient's fluid balance?

    a. Catheterise and measure hourly urine output.

    b. Ask the patient to urinate into a bottle and measure the resulting urine.

    c. Insert an arterial line and monitor BP trends.

    d. Give a fluid challenge and reassess BP and HR in 2 hours.

    e. Insert a central line and monitor central venous pressure (CVP) trends.

14. A 25-year-old male falls and sustains a distal radius fracture. After the cast is removed, he notices a lump in his wrist. How long does bone remodelling in an adult typically take?

    a. 1–3 years

    b. 3–5 years

    c. 5–7 years

    d. 7–10 years

    e. >10 years

15. Which of the following predisposes to thrombosis?

    a. Protein S overproduction

    b. Protein C overproduction

    c. Antithrombin III deficiency

    d. Antithrombin III overproduction

    e. Antiphospholipid deficiency

16. Which of the following disorders is *least* likely to be associated with the occurrence of a berry aneurysm in the Circle of Willis?

    a. Coarctation of the aorta

    b. Autosomal recessive polycystic kidney disease

    c. NF1

    d. Ehlers–Danlos syndrome

    e. Marfan's syndrome

17. Which of the following spirometry findings is characteristic of obstructive lung disease?

    a. Reduced vital capacity

    b. Increased forced expiratory volume in 1 second (FEV_1)/forced vital capacity (FVC) ratio

    c. Normal peak flow rate (peak expiratory flow rate [PEFR])

    d. Increased vital capacity

    e. Reduced FEV_1

18. Which of the following is true regarding lung cancer?

    a. Adenocarcinoma is usually located centrally within the lung parenchyma.

    b. Small-cell carcinoma is usually treated with chemotherapy.

    c. Without surgical resection, prognosis is good (>50% survival at 5 years).

    d. Squamous-cell lung cancer is often associated with paraneoplastic syndromes.

    e. Adenocarcinoma is always symptomatic.

19. Which of the following is true regarding prostate cancer?

    a. Most cancers are found in the transitional zone of the prostate.

    b. Most prostate cancers are transitional cell carcinomas.

    c. A prostate-specific antigen (PSA) level >8 ng/mL at any age is diagnostic of prostate carcinoma.

    d. Prostate cancer metastases to bone are sclerotic.

    e. Prostate cancer is the leading cause of death due to cancer in men.

20. Which of the following statements is true regarding acute pancreatitis?

    a. Hypocalcaemia occurs because of lipid saponification.

    b. A serum amylase level >100 U/L is diagnostic of acute pancreatitis.

    c. Antibiotics are always indicated in acute pancreatitis.

    d. Necrosis of the pancreas usually occurs within 24 hours of the onset of pain.

    e. Patients may require insulin therapy due to delta cell damage.

21. Which of the following is an example of an apoptosis-regulating gene?

    a. Bcl-2

    b. p53

    c. APC

    d. Ras

    e. ERB-1

22. Regarding Virchow's triad, which of the following is an example of venous stasis?

    a. Infection

    b. Malignancy

    c. Factor V Leiden

    d. Protein C deficiency

    e. Pregnancy

23. Regarding fungal infections in the immunosuppressed transplant patient, which of the following is true?

    a. *Cryptococcus* produces the carcinogen aflatoxin.

    b. *Pneumocystis carinii* is described as both a fungus and a protozoa.

    c. *Candida albicans* in the oesophagus is painless.

    d. *Histoplasma* is an invisible fungus.

    e. *Aspergillus* causes an immune reaction similar to TB.

24. Prostaglandins, leukotrienes, histamine and serotonin are all important inflammatory mediators released from which blood component?

    a. Platelets

    b. Macrophages

    c. Red blood cells

    d. B lymphocytes

    e. T lymphocytes

25. Which of the following statements is true regarding the aetiology of inflammation?

    a. Eosinophils predominate in typhoid and TB infections.

    b. Lymphocytes predominate in autoimmune disease.

    c. Neutrophils predominate in spirochaetal disease.

    d. Plasma cells predominate in bacterial infections.

    e. Macrophages predominate in viral infections.

26. Which of the following structures travels through the temporal bone?

    a. Mandibular branch of the trigeminal nerve

    b. Glossopharyngeal nerve

    c. Facial nerve

    d. Abducens nerve

    e. Optic nerve

27. A patient reports loss of taste sensation. Which branch of the facial nerve might be affected?

    a. Greater petrosal nerve

    b. Nerve to stapedius

    c. Lingual nerve

    d. Auricular nerve

    e. Chorda tympani

28. Following an injury to the right side of the head, a 35-year-old patient complains of double vision. On examination, his right eye is found turned outwards. It can move medially but not inferiorly or superiorly. You also notice ptosis and mydriasis. Which nerve is most likely to be affected?

    a. Optic

    b. Trochlear

    c. Abducens

    d. Nasociliary

    e. Oculomotor

29. A 25-year-old motorcyclist involved in a road traffic accident requires a chest drain for a right haemothorax. Which of the following statements is most likely to be true?

    a. A chest drain is usually inserted in the second intercostal space, at the midclavicular line.

    b. The endothoracic fascia is adherent to the inner thoracic cage between the innermost intercostal muscle and parietal pleura.

    c. The chest drain is directed under the rib above to avoid the neurovascular bundle on the superior edge of the rib.

    d. The neurovascular bundle runs between the external and internal intercostal muscles.

    e. The latissimus dorsi is passed through prior to traversing the intercostals.

30. Which of the following statements regarding the thymus is true?

    a. It is synonymous with the thyroid gland.

    b. It is derived from the second pair of pharyngeal pouches.

    c. It lies behind the trachea and oesophagus in the superior mediastinum.

    d. It contains lymphocytes and Hassall's corpuscles.

    e. Defects of the thymus lead to problems with thermoregulation.

31. A 45-year-old male injures his Achilles tendon playing squash. Which of the following muscles inserts into the Achilles tendon?

    a. Sartorius

    b. Semitendinosus

    c. Plantaris

    d. Gracilis

    e. Flexor digitorum longus

32. What important structure runs beneath the pterion?

    a. Pterygoid artery

    b. Middle meningeal artery

    c. Anterior cerebral artery

    d. Middle cerebral artery

    e. Superficial temporal artery

33. A 70-year-old male is undergoing an umbilical hernia repair. He has a left total hip replacement. Where should a diathermy plate ideally be placed?

    a. Over a bony prominence

    b. On a hair-free area prepared with an alcohol wipe

    c. Over an area bearing hair

    d. Over an area with a good blood supply

    e. Over a hip prosthesis

34. A 65-year-old male is seen in the preoperative assessment clinic prior to his elective total hip replacement. He is on warfarin for atrial fibrillation (AF). Which of the following statements is true of warfarin?

   a. It is a vitamin K antagonist.

   b. Its reversal agent is protamine.

   c. It acts directly on factor Xa in the clotting cascade.

   d. It does not require continuous monitoring.

   e. It binds to antithrombin III.

35. Which suture material would be best suited to repairing an artery?

   a. Vicryl®

   b. Vicryl Rapide™

   c. Monocryl™

   d. Prolene™

   e. Silk

36. What is the daily sodium requirement of a normal adult?

   a. 1 mmol/kg/L

   b. 2 mmol/kg/L

   c. 3 mmol/kg/L

   d. 4 mmol/kg/L

   e. 5 mmol/kg/L

37. By which route can fluid be administered to a patient?

   a. IV

   b. Subcutaneous

   c. Oral

   d. Intraosseous

   e. All of the above

38. In what state is the majority of calcium in the body found?

   a. Associated with citrate

   b. As hydroxyapatite

   c. Ionised in serum

   d. Bound to plasma proteins

   e. Associated with lactate

39. Which of the following molecules bind(s) to haemoglobin?

   a. CO_2

   b. Protons

   c. 2,3-DPG

   d. O_2

   e. All of the above

40. What is a normal CVP for a healthy adult?

   a. 0–10 mmHg

   b. 10–20 mmHg

   c. 20–30 mmHg

   d. 30–40 mmHg

   e. 40–50 mmHg

41. At thyroidectomy, the inferior thyroid artery is tied off. On waking, the patient notices some hoarseness of voice. Which nerve is most likely to have been affected?

   a. External laryngeal

   b. Recurrent laryngeal

   c. Glossopharyngeal

   d. Vagus

   e. Hypoglossal

42. A 54-year-old male presents with chronic diarrhoea. He has a colon-oscopy, during which biopsies are taken. These show non-caseating granulomata within the bowel wall. What is the diagnosis?

    a. Bowel cancer

    b. TB

    c. UC

    d. Crohn's disease

    e. Coeliac disease

43. You are dissecting out Calot's triangle during a laparoscopic cholecys-tectomy. What are the borders of Calot's triangle?

    a. Inferior edge of the liver, common hepatic duct, cystic duct

    b. Inferior edge of the liver, common hepatic artery, cystic duct

    c. Inferior edge of the liver, common hepatic artery, cystic artery

    d. Superior edge of the liver, common hepatic duct, cystic duct

    e. Superior edge of the liver, common hepatic artery, cystic artery

44. Which of the following is true regarding the small bowel?

    a. The whole of the small bowel is intra-peritoneal.

    b. All of the blood supply to the small bowel comes from the superior mesenteric artery.

    c. The small bowel mesentery runs from the duodenojejunal (DJ) flexure to the left iliac fossa.

    d. Small bowel can be identified on plain radiograph by the presence of valvulae conniventes.

    e. Small bowel can be identified at operation by the presence of taenia coli

45. Which of the following is the most common fatal cancer in women in the United Kingdom?

a. Breast carcinoma

b. Lung carcinoma

c. Ovarian carcinoma

d. Bowel carcinoma

e. None of the above

46. Which of the following is *not* part of MEN 1 syndrome?

a. Medullary thyroid carcinoma

b. Pancreatic islet cell tumour

c. Follicular thyroid carcinoma

d. Prolactinoma

e. Parathyroid carcinoma

47. Within what time of birth should meconium be passed by a healthy full-term neonate?

a. 12 hours

b. 24 hours

c. 48 hours

d. 5 days

e. 7 days

48. Which of the following does *not* affect the O_2–haemoglobin dissociation curve?

a. Temperature

b. CO_2

c. 2,3-DPG

d. Haemoglobin concentration

e. CO

49. A 35-year-old female falls from a 3 m high balcony and sustains a head injury. You assess her in A&E. Her eyes are open and she is making inappropriate speech. She flexes to pain. What is her GCS score?

a. 10

b. 11

c. 12

d. 13

e. 14

50. A 32-year-old who was an unrestrained passenger in a road traffic accident is brought into the ED triple immobilised and receiving high-flow O_2. She is talking, has an RR of 30 breaths/min, HR of 140 bpm and BP of 80/50 mmHg. Her trachea is central and air entry and percussion note are reduced in the left hemithorax. What is your first step in managing this patient?

a. Needle decompression of the left hemithorax in the third intercostal space, midclavicular line

b. Pericardiocentesis

c. Chest X-ray

d. Insertion of a surgical chest drain in the left hemithorax

e. Endotracheal intubation

MRCS Part A Paper 1

Mock Paper 5

Please select the single best answer from the five possible answers for each question.

Please answer all questions.

You have **45 minutes** to complete this paper.

1. Which of the following has alpha-blocking effects?

   a. Propranolol

   b. Labetalol

   c. Metoprolol

   d. Atenolol

   e. Timolol

2. Which of the following is a cause of aortic stenosis?

   a. Congenital bicuspid valve

   b. Rheumatic fever

   c. Hypertension

   d. Age-related calcification

   e. All of the above

3. Which of the following is a neuroendocrine tumour of the pancreas?

   a. Teratoma

   b. Adenocarcinoma

   c. Lymphoma

   d. Gastrinoma

   e. None of the above

4. Which of these structures is found in the trans-pyloric plane?

   a. Root of the coeliac trunk

   b. Lower pole of the kidneys

   c. Neck of the pancreas

   d. L3 vertebra

   e. Third part of the duodenum

5. A female with recurrent peptic ulcers is found to have Zollinger–Ellison syndrome, resulting in the production of excess stomach acid. What mechanism is responsible for this acid overproduction?

   a. Gastrin release from a neuroendocrine tumour

   b. Increased vagal parasympathetic excitability

   c. Cholecystokinin release following a fatty meal

   d. Stomach irritation due to an adenocarcinoma

   e. Excess production of pepsinogen by chief cells

6. A 70-year-old male is diagnosed with oesophageal adenocarcinoma. Which of the following statements is true regarding oesophageal cancer?

   a. Smoking and alcohol use are the main risk factors for oesophageal adenocarcinoma.

   b. Squamous-cell carcinoma is more common than adenocarcinoma in the United Kingdom.

   c. Barrett's oesophagus is an early form of oesophageal cancer.

   d. Adenocarcinoma is most commonly situated in the lower third of the oesophagus.

   e. Those with Barrett's oesophagus are at high risk for developing squamous-cell carcinoma.

7. A 65-year-old smoker presents with an acutely pale, cold and painful left foot. Where would you palpate for foot pulses?

   a. Dorsum of foot, medial to the extensor hallucis longus and anterior border of the medial malleolus

   b. Dorsum of foot, medial to the flexor hallucis longus and anterior border of the lateral malleolus

   c. Dorsum of foot, lateral to the flexor hallucis longus and posterior border of the lateral malleolus

   d. Dorsum of foot, just lateral to the extensor hallucis longus and posterior border of the medial malleolus

   e. Dorsum of foot, lateral to the flexor hallucis brevis and posterior border to the medial malleolus

8. A 60-year-old female develops pain when attempting to raise her left shoulder. On examination, you find she has a great deal of pain at 60–120 degrees of abduction. Which rotator cuff muscle is most likely to be affected?

   a. Supraspinatus

   b. Infraspinatus

   c. Teres major

   d. Teres minor

   e. Subscapularis

9. A 30-year-old male is brought into the ED with a head injury. His mean arterial pressure (MAP) should be kept at what level?

   a. 30 mmHg

   b. 40 mmHg

   c. 50 mmHg

   d. 60 mmHg

   e. 70 mmHg

10. You are called to the ward to prescribe fluids post-operatively to a 77-year-old male who has undergone an endovascular aortic aneurysm repair. What are the maintenance requirements for fluid in the average 70 kg male?

    a. 1.0–1.2 L water and 40–50 mmol/L sodium; 20–30 mmol/L potassium

    b. 1.5–2.5 L water and 30–60 mmol/L sodium; 30–40 mmol/L potassium

    c. 1.5–2.5 L water and 50–100 mmol/L sodium; 40–80 mmol/L potassium

    d. 1.5–2.5 L water and 130–150 mmol/l sodium; 40–80 mmol/L potassium

    e. 1.5–2.5 L water and 130–150 mmol/L sodium; 80–100 mmol/L potassium

11. A 55-year-old female presents with an acutely swollen left leg following her recent trip to South Africa. She is a lifelong smoker and takes hormone replacement therapy. While on holiday, she was bitten by an insect on her left foot. You find no erythema on examination. What is the most likely cause of her symptoms?

   a. Necrotising fasciitis

   b. Cellulitis

   c. Lymphoedema

   d. Deep vein thrombosis

   e. Necrobiosis lipoidica

12. A 20-year-old female falls from her horse and sustains a distal radius fracture. What type of bone is initially formed in the reparative phase of fracture healing?

   a. Compact

   b. Woven

   c. Lamellar

   d. Trabecular

   e. Spongy

13. Which of the following organisms is most likely to cause meningitis in neonates?

   a. *Neisseria meningitides*

   b. *Haemophilus influenzae*

   c. *Staphylococcus aureus*

   d. *Mycobacterium tuberculosis*

   e. *Escherichia coli*

14. Which of the following organisms is most likely to cause a breast abscess in a non-lactating female?

    a. *Staphylococcus aureus*

    b. *Streptococcus viridans*

    c. *Staphylococcus epidermidis*

    d. *Bacteroides fragilis*

    e. *Lactobacillus acidophilus*

15. Which of the following cytological features identifies malignant cells?

    a. Nuclear pleomorphism

    b. Well differentiated cells

    c. Low nuclear/cytoplasmic ratio

    d. Hypochromatism

    e. Low number of mitoses

16. Regarding Virchow's triad, which of the following is an example of a hypercoagulable state?

    a. Prolonged anaesthesia

    b. Poor nutrition

    c. Poor mobility

    d. Smoking

    e. Use of a tourniquet

17. Which of the following statements regarding statistical data is true?

    a. Sex and ethnicity are examples of ordinal data.

    b. The mode is the middle value in a data set.

    c. Weight and height are discrete variables.

    d. Standard deviation is a measure of data spread.

    e. GCS score and age are examples of nominal data.

18. Regarding hypersensitivity reactions, which of the following statements is true?

    a. Myasthenia gravis is an example of a type IV reaction.
    b. Acute glomerulonephritis is an example of a type III reaction.
    c. A type III reaction is antibody mediated.
    d. Type V reactions are mediated by T lymphocytes.
    e. Anaphylaxis is an example of a type II reaction.

19. Which of the following statements is true regarding post-operative wound infection?

    a. Preoperative shaving can increase the incidence of wound infection.
    b. In immunocompromised patients, wound infection is most commonly fungal.
    c. The incidence of post-operative VTE disease correlates with wound infection rates.
    d. Immunocompromised patients always mount a systemic response to wound infections.
    e. None of the above.

20. Which of the following statements regarding chronic inflammation is true?

    a. Granulomatous disease is not an example.
    b. The predominant cell type is polymorphonuclear.
    c. There is evidence of healing with angiogenesis.
    d. Tissue destruction is completely halted.
    e. Scarring involves laying down type IV collagen fibres.

21. Which of the following statements regarding the bones of the skull is true?

   a. The occipital bone transmits the vestibulocochlear nerve.

   b. The sphenoid bone transmits the facial nerve.

   c. The temporal bone transmits the abducens nerve.

   d. The petrous temporal bone transmits the lesser petrosal nerve.

   e. The frontal bone transmits the zygomatic nerve.

22. You examine a patient after a right parotidectomy. On examining his facial nerve, he is unable to bear his teeth to you. Which branch of the facial nerve is most likely to have been damaged?

   a. Mandibular

   b. Zygomatic

   c. Buccal

   d. Temporal

   e. Cervical

23. A 23-year-old male is hit in the eye with a cricket ball. You suspect a blowout fracture of the orbit. Which eye movements are most likely to be affected?

   a. Lateral

   b. Downward and medial

   c. Upward and medial

   d. Medial

   e. Downward and lateral

24. A 3-year-old male attends A&E with his mother who is concerned that he has inhaled a piece of Lego®. Which of the following statements is true?

   a. The trachea bifurcates at the level of T6.

   b. As the left main bronchus is larger in diameter and forms less of an angle with the trachea than the right main bronchus, foreign bodies usually lodge there.

   c. The angle of Louis is where the clavicle joins the sternum.

   d. The left lung has three lobes: upper, middle and lower.

   e. The lung under the anterior surface of the left chest wall is predominantly upper lobe.

25. Which of the following statements is true regarding the aorta?

   a. The ascending aorta has no branches.

   b. The descending aorta is related anteriorly to the left main bronchus.

   c. The thoracic aorta runs in both the inferior and superior mediastina.

   d. The descending aorta has direct anterior intercostal arterial branches.

   e. The descending aorta crosses the diaphragm into the abdomen at T10.

26. During a mastectomy, care is taken to ensure adequate haemostasis. Which of the following statements regarding the blood supply of the breast is true?

    a. The major arterial supply is directly from the thoracic aorta.

    b. The medial breast is supplied by branches from the anterior intercostal arteries.

    c. Deep perforating vessels pierce the pectoralis major and are derived from the thyrocervical trunk.

    d. The epigastric arteries supply the rectus muscle and are all derived from the internal thoracic artery.

    e. None of the above.

27. A 35-year-old female presents with abdominal pain. Which of the following structures is retroperitoneal?

    a. Caecum

    b. Appendix

    c. Second part of the duodenum

    d. Tail of the pancreas

    e. Ovaries

28. A 55-year-old male sustains a distal fibular fracture while running. How many fascial compartments are in the leg?

    a. Two

    b. Three

    c. Four

    d. Five

    e. Six

29. A 16-year-old male is hit by a cricket ball in the temporal region of the head. The weak junction between bones in the temporal region is called the 'pterion'. How many bones form this weak junction?

a. Two

b. Three

c. Four

d. Five

e. Six

30. During most surgical procedures, diathermy is used for haemostasis. Which of the following statements is true?

a. The active and return electrodes are in the same instrument in monopolar diathermy.

b. The most common cause of accidental burns is misapplication of the diathermy plate.

c. Diathermy uses low-frequency direct current.

d. Alcohol skin preparations reduce the risks of surgical infection and fire.

e. The presence of an implantable cardioverter-defibrillator is an absolute contraindication to all diathermy.

31. Which of the following organs is/are involved in acid–base balance?

a. Lungs

b. Blood

c. Kidneys

d. Liver

e. All of the above

32. A 70-year-old female comes into A&E with a posterior dislocation of her right total hip replacement. You decide to try and reduce it in A&E and administer a benzodiazepine to sedate the patient. What agent reverses benzodiazepines?

    a. Naloxone

    b. Intralipid®

    c. Morphine

    d. Flumazenil

    e. Protamine

33. A patient with AF is assessed preoperatively for an elective laparoscopic cholecystectomy. Which of these is an example of a non-invasive cardiac test?

    a. Trans-thoracic echocardiogram

    b. BP monitoring via an arterial line

    c. Pulmonary artery catheter

    d. Bronchoscopy

    e. Endotracheal intubation

34. A 45-year-old female presents with epigastric pain and is diagnosed with acute pancreatitis. As part of VTE prophylaxis, you prescribe low-molecular-weight heparin (LMWH). Which of the following statements is true?

    a. It acts on clotting factors II, VII, IX and X.

    b. It is usually administered in an oral preparation.

    c. Protamine is the reversal agent.

    d. It is a direct factor Xa inhibitor.

    e. It requires daily serum level monitoring.

35. A 35-year-old type 1 diabetic is on dialysis awaiting a transplant. Which of the following is an indication for haemofiltration/ haemodialysis?

   a. Hypokalaemia (K+ <3.5 mmol/L)

   b. Uraemia (urea >10 mmol/L)

   c. Creatinine clearance <60 mL/min

   d. Refractory pulmonary oedema

   e. None of the above

36. Which of the following is a cause of hyponatraemia?

   a. SIADH

   b. Nephrotic syndrome

   c. Diarrhoea

   d. TUR of the prostate syndrome

   e. All of the above

37. Which of the following would be the most accurate way of assessing ventilation?

   a. Pulse oximetry

   b. Sphygmomanometry

   c. Peak flow measurement

   d. Capnography

   e. Bronchoscopy

38. A 70-year-old male has complications following an elective TUR of the prostate. He is taken back to theatre because of bleeding on two separate occasions. Once he is extubated and recovering on the intensive care unit, which drug should you consider starting this patient on?

    a. Statin

    b. Antiplatelet

    c. Proton pump inhibitor

    d. Diuretic

    e. None of the above

39. Which of the following is true regarding the large bowel?

    a. The rectum is the most distensible part of the large bowel.

    b. Appendices epiploicae are features of the large bowel rather than the small bowel.

    c. The large bowel can be identified on plan X-ray by the presence of lines crossing the whole diameter of the bowel.

    d. The rectum is the most common area of ischaemia due to its poor blood supply.

    e. The most common malignancy of the large bowel is lymphoma.

40. Which of the following is most likely to result from an increase in PTH level?

    a. Reduced calcium reabsorption in the kidney

    b. Reduced calcium absorption in the intestine

    c. Increased vitamin D activation in the kidney

    d. Inhibition of osteoclastic activity

    e. Reduced phosphate excretion in the kidney

41. A patient with pancreatitis develops a pseudocyst within the lesser sac. Which of the following structures lies directly in front of the pseudocyst?

    a. Pancreas

    b. Stomach

    c. Duodenum

    d. Splenic artery

    e. Liver

42. A patient notices a persistent lump in their neck. A biopsy is taken showing the presence of Reed–Sternberg cells. What is the diagnosis?

    a. Hodgkin's lymphoma

    b. Non-Hodgkin's lymphoma

    c. TB

    d. Acute lymphoblastic leukaemia

    e. Chronic lymphocytic leukaemia

43. Which of the following is a possible feature of hypothyroidism?

    a. Hypercalcaemia

    b. Palmar erythema

    c. Brisk reflexes

    d. Reduced appetite

    e. AF

44. A patient is admitted with raised potassium. Which of the following drugs is most likely to be responsible?

    a. Furosemide

    b. Ramipril

    c. Calcium supplements

    d. Bendroflumethiazide

    e. Aspirin

45. A patient is brought to the ED following a major trauma. They are given 15 units of packed red cells in a 24-hour period. Which of the following metabolic disturbances are they at risk of?

   a. Hypocalcaemia

   b. Hyperkalaemia

   c. Hypomagnesaemia

   d. Hypokalaemia

   e. All of the above

46. One of your patients has an ECG. The trace appears as a sine wave. What is the most appropriate initial treatment?

   a. Amiodarone

   b. Calcium gluconate

   c. Glyceryl trinitrate spray

   d. Atropine

   e. Adenosine

47. You are concerned about the possibility of lymphatic spread in a patient with ovarian cancer. Which group of lymph nodes do the ovaries drain to?

   a. Inguinal

   b. Superior rectal

   c. Pre-sacral

   d. Renal hilar

   e. Para-aortic

48. You see a male in clinic who is thought to have obstructive jaundice. Which of the following is a feature of obstructive jaundice?

a. Increased unconjugated bilirubin in serum

b. Increased urobilinogen excreted in stool

c. Decreased urobilinogen excreted in urine

d. Decreased bilirubin in serum

e. Reduction in serum alanine transaminase (ALT)

49. A patient is brought to the ED with extensive burns from a fire. Which of the following is most likely to be a feature of a full-thickness burn?

a. Erythematous surface

b. Loss of skin sensation

c. Skin blistering

d. Moist skin

e. Skin hypersensitivity

50. Which of the following is included as part of the Child–Pugh assessment of chronic liver disease severity?

a. Serum bilirubin

b. Prothrombin time

c. Presence of ascites

d. Presence of encephalopathy

e. All of the above

MRCS Part A Paper 2

Mock Paper 6

Please answer all questions.

You have **45 minutes** to complete this paper.

Theme: fluid balance

Please answer each question with one of the following options. Each option may be used once, more than once or not at all.

a. Hyperchloraemic acidosis

b. Hartmann's solution

c. 0.9% saline solution

d. Gelofusin

e. 0.45% dextrose/saline solution

f. 5% dextrose solution

g. Hyponatraemia

h. 40–80 mmol/day

i. 50–100 mmol/day

j. 20–30 mL/kg/day

k. 30–40 mL/kg/day

l. 60–80 mL/kg/day

1. Which fluid is advised as first line for use in fluid resuscitation of an adult?

2. What are patients at risk of if 0.9% saline solution is the only fluid therapy used?

3. Which fluid can cause hyponatraemia if given alone in large volumes as an IV resuscitation fluid?

4. What is the daily fluid requirement for the average 70 kg male?

5. What is the daily sodium requirement for the average 70 kg male?

Theme: pain control

Please answer each question with one of the following options. Each option may be used once, more than once or not at all.

a. 2 mg/kg

b. 3 mg/kg

c. 7 mg/kg

d. Paracetamol

e. Non-steroidal anti-inflammatory drugs (NSAIDs)

f. Spinal anaesthesia

g. Peripheral nerve block

h. Opiates

i. Reduce the background infusion

j. Reduce the bolus dose

6. During a knee arthroscopy in a 45-year-old male, local anaesthetic is injected into the skin prior to port insertion. What maximum dose of plain lignocaine is used?

7. A 35-year-old diabetic has an arteriovenous fistula formed in the forearm under local anaesthetic. What maximum dose of plain bupivacaine is used?

8. Following an elective total knee replacement, a 55-year-old male is hypotensive and oliguric on the ward. He does not have patient-controlled analgesia (PCA). What else can cause this?

9. Following a femoro-femoral crossover bypass graft insertion, a 65-year-old female is drowsy on the ward. What analgesic may have caused this?

10. A patient is sent back from recovery following a right total knee replacement with PCA. They have a background infusion and bolus dose with a 5-minute lockout period. The patient is very drowsy. What should you do?

Theme: head injury

Please answer each question with one of the following options. Each option may be used once, more than once or not at all.

a. Glasgow score

b. Airway/C-spine immobilisation

c. Subarachnoid haemorrhage

d. C-spine immobilisation

e. GCS

f. Head CT scan

g. Magnetic resonance imaging (MRI) of the head

h. Extradural haemorrhage

i. Intubation

j. Skull X-ray

k. Secondary brain injury

l. Primary brain injury

11. A 30-year-old male is involved in a road traffic accident and sustains a head injury. What is the first thing you do in your initial assessment?

12. A 35-year-old male is assaulted and sustains a head injury. How do you assess his level of consciousness?

13. A 45-year-old female falls at home and is brought in to ED by her partner. She is intoxicated and her partner reports that there was no initial loss of consciousness. However, in the last hour she has become drowsy and vomited twice. After a full clinical examination, what is indicated next?

14. A 20-year-old male is hit in the head with a tennis ball. Initially he appears fine, however, 4 hours later, his friends bring him into the ED with a reduced level of consciousness. What do you suspect is the cause?

15. A 65-year-old male falls down the stairs at home. He is unconscious on arrival in the ED and after initial assessment is intubated and ventilated to maintain good oxygenation and normocarbia. What does this help prevent?

Theme: compartment syndrome

Please answer each question with one of the following options. Each option may be used once, more than once or not at all.

a. Pallor

b. Paraesthesia

c. Pain

d. 40 mmHg

e. 30 mmHg

f. 50 mmHg

g. Split the cast

h. Fasciotomy

i. Muscle necrosis

j. Volkmann's ischaemic contracture

k. Four incisions

l. Two incisions

16. In a conscious patient, what is the most reliable clinical feature of compartment syndrome?

17. Fasciotomy is indicated when the pressure difference between the diastolic BP and compartment pressure reaches what?

18. A 30-year-old male is on the ward 6 hours post intramedullary nailing of a right tibial fracture. His has a backslab plaster cast on and is complaining of pain in the same leg. After initial examination, you are suspicious of compartment syndrome. What should your very first step be?

19. What is the long-term consequence of delayed fasciotomy in compartment syndrome?

20. How many incisions do you need to open all four compartments in the leg?

Theme: fracture management

Please answer each question with one of the following options. Each option may be used once, more than once or not at all.

a. Closed reduction and fixation with a cast

b. Functional bracing

c. Skin traction

d. Open reduction and internal fixation

e. External fixation

f. Percutaneous fixation with Kirschner wires

g. Arthroplasty

h. Hemiarthroplasty

i. Skeletal traction

j. Skin traction

k. Thomas splint

21. An 85-year-old female with multiple co-morbidities sustains a minimally displaced distal radius fracture of her non-dominant hand following a fall. How would you manage this?

22. A fit and well 30-year-old male sustains a distal radius fracture with volar displacement of his dominant hand. How would you manage this?

23. An 8-year-old male falls from his bicycle and sustains a minimally displaced supracondylar fracture, with no neurovascular compromise. How would you manage this?

24. An 89-year-old male who mobilises with a frame at home sustains an intracapsular neck-of-femur fracture. How would you manage this?

25. A 40-year-old male sustains open comminuted tibia and fibula fractures during a road traffic accident. How would you treat these?

Theme: arthritis

Please answer each question with one of the following options. Each option may be used once, more than once or not at all.

a. Gram stain

b. India ink stain

c. Joint aspiration

d. X-ray

e. Bloods and blood cultures

f. Joint-space narrowing and osteophyte formation

g. Joint-space narrowing and osteopenia

h. Pencil-in-cup deformity

i. Rheumatoid arthritis

j. Osteoarthritis

k. Osteoporosis

26. A 65-year-old female presents with an acutely painful, swollen and hot right knee. She underwent right total knee replacement 5 months ago. She is pyrexial. What is the most important investigation that should be done?

27. A 45-year-old IV drug user presents with a swollen, painful and hot left hip. She is pyrexial. You arrange an USS that reveals an effusion. You ask the radiologist to aspirate it and send the sample for what?

28. A 65-year-old female complains of right hip pain, which is worse on weight bearing, with increasing stiffness of the joint. She is over-weight and has a medical history of type 2 diabetes, hypertension and high cholesterol. What is the most likely cause of her symptoms?

29. A 70-year-old female had a right total hip replacement 18 months ago for osteoarthritis. Having recovered well, she would now like her left hip replaced for the same problem. What X-ray changes would you expect to see on the left hip?

30. A 35-year-old female presents with symptoms of tingling and numbness in her right hand, particularly over her thumb and index finger. On further questioning, she also reports pain in the small joints, especially her knuckles, which have started to swell. What X-ray changes would you expect to see?

Theme: groin and testicular lumps

Please answer each question with one of the following options. Each option may be used once, more than once or not at all.

a. Hydrocele

b. Teratoma

c. Varicocele

d. Indirect inguinal hernia

e. Femoral hernia

f. Lymphadenopathy

g. Testicular torsion

h. Epididymitis

i. Torted hydatid cyst

31. A 65-year-old male attends clinic with swelling of his left testicle. He complains of a dragging sensation on that side and has noticed blood in his urine over the past few weeks. On further questioning, he mentions that he has been taking painkillers for discomfort in his left flank and that he has recently lost 6 kg in weight. What is the most likely diagnosis?

32. A 25-year-old male who has recently been catheterised presents with a painful right testicle. The pain has increased gradually over the past week. On examination, you find it swollen and exquisitely tender. The cremasteric reflex is present. What is the most likely diagnosis?

33. A 40-year-old female has noticed a lump in her right groin that varies in size throughout the day and is normally smaller at night. The lump is situated below and lateral to the pubic tubercle. It has no cough impulse. What is the most likely diagnosis?

34. A 40-year-old male who is on peritoneal dialysis presents to A&E with a swollen right testicle. It is not tender to palpation and does not extend into the groin. The swelling can be transilluminated. What is the most likely diagnosis?

35. A 13-year-old male complains of pain in his left testicle that came on suddenly a few hours ago. On examination, you find it is tender. The cremasteric reflex is absent. What is the most likely diagnosis?

Theme: abdominal surgery

Please answer each question with one of the following options. Each option may be used once, more than once or not at all.

a. Appendicitis

b. Acute cholecystitis

c. Meckel's diverticulitis

d. Appendices epiploicae

e. Taenia coli

f. Biliary colic

g. Chronic pancreatitis

h. Perforated duodenal ulcer

i. Acute cholangitis

j. Acute pancreatitis

36. An 8-year-old male undergoes laparoscopy for acute abdominal pain. During the operation, you see an inflamed, blind-ended tube on the anti-mesenteric surface of ileum. What is the most likely pathology?

37. What are the small pouches of fat-filled peritoneum associated with the colon and upper rectum called?

38. A 36-year-old female with known gallstones presents with right upper quadrant pain. She is febrile and has raised inflammatory markers. Amylase and liver function biochemistry are normal. What is the most likely pathology?

39. A 49-year-old alcoholic presents with weight loss and floating stools that will not flush away. What is the most likely pathology?

40. A 36-year-old female with known gallstones presents with right upper quadrant pain, pale urine and dark stools. She is febrile and has raised inflammatory markers. Her serum amylase is normal. What is the most likely pathology?

Theme: rectal bleeding

Please answer each question with one of the following options. Each option may be used once, more than once or not at all.

a. Diverticular disease

b. Haemorrhoids

c. Anal fissure

d. Duodenal ulcer

e. Rectal adenocarcinoma

f. Inflammatory bowel disease

g. Intestinal ischaemia

h. Peptic ulcer

i. Diverticular disease

41. An 80-year-old male is brought to A&E with severe abdominal pain and PR bleeding. The pain seems out of proportion to your clinical findings. He has a history of AF, for which he is on aspirin. What is the most likely diagnosis?

42. A 25-year-old male with constipation has noticed blood on the toilet paper after opening his bowels. For the past week, defaecation has been extremely painful. He says it feels 'like passing glass'. What is the most likely diagnosis?

43. A 22-year-old male is seen in clinic with a history of diarrhoea, intermittent abdominal pain and rectal bleeding. He has noticed that his stool contains both blood and mucus. He takes NSAIDs for arthralgia. What is the most likely diagnosis?

44. A 32-year-old female in her third trimester of pregnancy attends the colorectal clinic. She has noticed fresh blood and a small amount of mucous on the toilet paper. There is no blood in the toilet pan or mixed in with the stool. She has been suffering from itching around the anus. What is the most likely diagnosis?

45. A 75-year-old male on long-term steroids presents to A&E with heavy PR bleeding. The blood is bright red and is passed even when not defaecating. He has a history of intermittent epigastric pain and is tender in this region. What is the most likely diagnosis?

Theme: suture materials

Please answer each question with one of the following options. Each option may be used once, more than once or not at all.

a. Sorbsan® dressing

b. Monofilament, dissolvable suture

c. Braided, non-dissolvable suture

d. Monofilament, non-dissolvable suture

e. Surgical clip

f. Steri-Strip™

g. Skin glue

h. Deep-tension suture

i. Reverse-cutting needle

j. Round-bodied needle

46. Which suture material/instrument is typically most appropriate for surgical drain fixation?

47. Which suture material/instrument is typically most appropriate for brachiocephalic anastomosis in arteriovenous fistula formation?

48. Which suture material/instrument is typically most appropriate for skin closure in a primary inguinal hernia repair?

49. Which suture material/instrument is typically most appropriate for closing a pre-tibial laceration?

50. Which suture material/instrument is typically most appropriate to close the skin of a full-length midline laparotomy incision?

MRCS Part A Paper 2

Mock Paper 7

Please answer all questions.

You have **45 minutes** to complete this paper.

Theme: trauma assessment and management

Please answer each question with one of the following options. Each option may be used once, more than once or not at all.

- a. Urgent thoracotomy
- b. Chest drain insertion, left
- c. Chest drain insertion, right
- d. Pericardiocentesis
- e. Needle decompression, left thorax
- f. Needle decompression, right thorax
- g. Endotracheal intubation
- h. Bag-mask ventilation
- i. Nasopharyngeal airway
- j. O_2
- k. Head CT scan

1. A 45-year-old male is brought to the ED following a high-speed vehicle crash. His airway is patent and self-maintained and he is receiving O_2. He has an RR of 30 breaths/min, with reduced air entry and dullness to percussion on the left. His HR is 100/min and BP is 110/70mmHg. What is the most appropriate next management step?

2. An 18-year-old female has been knocked off her bicycle, sustaining severe head injuries. She has a GCS score of 5 and bruising around both eyes. She is receiving O_2, has an RR of 6 breaths/min and O_2 saturations of 80% on O_2. She has equal air entry bilaterally on auscultation. No anaesthetist is available. What is the most appropriate first management step?

3. A 60-year-old male has fallen from a first-floor balcony. He is on O_2, has a patent airway, an RR of 28 breaths/min, hyperresonance to percussion in his left chest and his trachea is deviated to the right. What is the most appropriate next management step?

4. A 75-year-old female has been hit by a car on a pedestrian crossing. She is asking about her husband who was also hit. She appears confused. Her RR is 20 breaths/min and O_2 saturations are 90% on air. What is the most appropriate first management step?

5. A 20-year-old motorcyclist has an intercostal drain inserted for a left-sided haemothorax and 1600 mL drains instantly. He has IV access and is receiving O_2. What is the next most appropriate management step?

Theme: ABG sampling

Please answer each question with one of the following options. *Each option may be used only once.*

All samples are on room air.

a. pH 7.29; PaCO$_2$, 3.2; pO$_2$, 18.4; glucose, 5.6; lactate, 9.2

b. pH 7.13; PaCO$_2$, 6.5; pO$_2$, 7.9; glucose, 5.9; lactate, 1.2

c. pH 7.35; PaCO$_2$, 4.2; pO$_2$, 14.1; glucose, 6.3; lactate, 1.1

d. pH 6.95; PaCO$_2$, 3.2; pO$_2$, 18.0; glucose, 32.0; lactate, 0.8

e. pH 7.55; PaCO$_2$, 3.2; pO$_2$, 18.4; glucose, 32.0; lactate, 0.8

f. pH 7.47; PaCO$_2$, 3.0; pO$_2$, 20.0; glucose, 6.1; lactate, 1.0

g. pH 7.35; PaCO$_2$, 4.0; pO$_2$, 7.8; glucose, 18.0; lactate, 0.8

h. pH 7.29; PaCO$_2$, 3.2; pO$_2$, 13.8; glucose, 9.2; lactate, 3.4

i. Buerger's test

j. Palmar anastomosis test

k. Allen's test

6. Before undertaking radial artery blood sampling, collateral blood supply to the hand via the ulnar artery should be assessed. What is the name of this test?

7. A 64-year-old alcoholic presents extremely unwell with acute epigastric pain, radiating to his back. His serum amylase is 2400 U/L. Which set of ABG results is most likely to be his?

8. A 21-year-old asthmatic presents with increased shortness of breath that has not responded to nebulisers. He is tired and has little air entry on auscultation. Which set of ABG results is most likely to be his?

9. A 16-year-old presents extremely unwell, with weight loss, polyuria and polydipsia. Which set of ABG results is the most likely to belong to this patient?

10. A 71-year-old with known AF, for which she does not take warfarin, collapses with acute abdominal pain. Which set of ABG results is most likely to be hers?

Theme: carotid disease

Please answer each question with one of the following options. Each option may be used once, more than once or not at all.

a. Anticoagulation

b. Antiplatelet therapy

c. Conservative management

d. Right carotid endarterectomy

e. Left carotid endarterectomy

f. Carotid duplex scan

g. Magnetic resonance angiography (MRA) scan

h. Digital subtraction angiography (DSA) scan

i. CT angiography scan

j. Atherosclerosis

k. Carotid body tumour

l. Fibromuscular dysplasia

11. A 70-year-old female presents with neurological symptoms and carotid artery stenosis is diagnosed. What is the most common cause of this?

12. A 60-year-old male had symptoms of amaurosis fugax, which have now resolved. Following a full clinical examination, what is the standard imaging used to assess the carotids?

13. A 75-year-old female suffers from TIAs that affect her right arm. She has 90% stenosis in the left carotid and 20% in the right. How would you manage this patient?

14. A 65-year-old male suffers transient neurological symptoms affecting his left arm. He is found to have 80% stenosis in the right carotid artery and 70% in the left. How would you manage this patient?

15. A 75-year-old male suffers TIAs and is found to have AF. Investigations show he also has 60% carotid artery stenosis on the left and 40% on the right. What should be considered in the management of this patient?

Theme: fracture healing

Please answer each question with one of the following options. Each option may be used once, more than once or not at all.

a. Infection

b. Soft tissue interposition

c. Avascular necrosis

d. Hypertrophic non-union

e. Atrophic non-union

f. Delayed union

g. Malunion

h. Amputation

16. A fracture of the humeral shaft heals with considerable shortening and with the distal limb externally rotated. What is the most likely pathology?

17. A fracture of the tibial shaft is fixed with an intermedullary nail. The patient is a smoker and the fracture has failed to heal after 6 weeks. What is the most likely pathology?

18. A compound fracture of the distal tibia/fibula fails to heal following infection. There is abundant callus formation on the X-ray. What is the most likely pathology?

19. A scaphoid fracture fails to heal and this has resulted in chronic pain. What is the most likely pathology?

20. A fracture of the shaft of the humerus fails to heal in an older diabetic patient. There is a lack of callus formation on the X-ray. What is the most likely pathology?

Theme: hernias

Please answer each question with one of the following options. Each option may be used once, more than once or not at all.

a. Indirect inguinal hernia

b. Direct inguinal hernia

c. Femoral hernia

d. Ilioinguinal nerve

e. Iliohypogastric nerve

f. Lateral cutaneous nerve of the thigh

g. Medial cutaneous nerve of the thigh

h. Testicular artery

i. Testicular vein

j. Vas deferens

21. A 45-year-old builder presents with a groin lump. On examination, you find the lump above and lateral to the pubic tubercle with a cough impulse. If you reduce the lump and place your hand over the internal ring, the lump does not reappear on coughing. What is the most likely diagnosis?

22. At open hernia repair, you find that the hernia sac lies lateral to the inferior epigastric artery. What is the most likely diagnosis?

23. A 56-year-old female has a groin lump. On examination, you find she has a lump with a cough impulse below and medial to the pubic tubercle. What is the most likely diagnosis?

24. A 76-year-old male undergoes elective open left inguinal hernia repair. He presents several months later with a reduction in size of his left testicle. Which structure has most likely been damaged?

25. A 72-year-old male undergoes elective open right inguinal hernia repair. He complains of numbness of the right medial thigh and scrotal skin. Which structure has most likely been damaged?

Theme: spinal trauma

Please answer each question with one of the following options. Each option may be used once, more than once or not at all.

a. Neurogenic shock

b. Spinal shock

c. C-spine immobilisation

d. Neck collar

e. X-ray of the spine

f. CT scan of the spine

g. MRI of the spine

h. Stable fracture

i. Unstable fracture

j. Nuclear medicine bone scan

26. A 20-year-old male is violently assaulted and sustains significant head and spinal injuries. He has marked bruising and lacerations at the T10–12 level and, on examination, you find he has flaccid areflexia below this level and loss of anal tone. What is the diagnosis?

27. A 15-year-old female falls from her horse and sustains an unstable fracture of the T2. She is hypotensive and bradycardic. What is the diagnosis?

28. A 30-year-old male falls from a ladder while cleaning first-storey windows. He walks into the ED holding his head and complaining of neck pain. What is your first step?

29. A 40-year-old female is involved in a road traffic accident and sustains a unilateral facet dislocation at C6. How would you define this fracture's stability?

30. A 19-year-old male sustains a back injury playing rugby. He has no notable neurology but is complaining of severe pain around his lumbar spine. Initial X-rays are unhelpful in excluding serious pathology. What should you do next?

Theme: nutrition

Please answer each question with one of the following options. Each option may be used once, more than once or not at all.

a. Unintentional weight loss >10% in 3–6 months

b. Inadequate oral intake for 5 days or more

c. Poor absorptive capacity

d. Prevent bacterial translocation

e. Parenteral

f. Enteral

g. Prevent multi-organ failure

h. Small bowel fistula

i. Percutaneous gastrostomy

j. Peripherally inserted central catheter line

k. NG tube

l. Nasojejunal (NJ) tube

m. BMI <19 kg/m^2

31. How is malnutrition defined?

32. Which feeding route preserves the integrity of the intestinal wall?

33. Why is it important to preserve intestinal lumen barrier function?

34. When might enteral feeding be contraindicated?

35. What is the preferred method of delivering enteral feeds required for more than 2 months?

Theme: local anaesthesia

Please answer each question with one of the following options. Each option may be used once, more than once or not at all.

a. 12 mL

b. 50 mL

c. 4 mL

d. 420 mL

e. 42 mL

f. 20 mL

g. 0.5% bupivacaine with adrenaline

h. 0.5% bupivacaine

i. Intralipid®

j. Naloxone

36. A 1-year-old male weighing 10 kg undergoes inguinal hernia repair. What is the maximum volume of 0.5% plain bupivacaine that you may infiltrate into the skin?

37. A 40-year-old female weighing 60 kg has a lipoma removed under local anaesthetic. What is the maximum volume of 1% lignocaine with adrenaline that you can use?

38. A 35-year-old male weighing 80 kg requires a chest drain for a haemothorax. What is the maximum volume of 2% plain lignocaine that you can use?

39. A 10-year-old male traps his finger in a door and requires a nail bed repair. What is the most appropriate local anaesthetic for the ring block?

40. What is the antidote for local-anaesthetic sensitivity?

Theme: statistics

Please answer each question with one of the following options. Each option may be used once, more than once or not at all.

a. Sensitivity

b. Specificity

c. Odds ratio

d. Relative risk

e. Negative predictive value

f. Positive predictive value

g. False negative

h. False positive

i. Incidence

j. Prevalence

41. You develop a new test for appendicitis. You discover that the test correctly identifies 86% of those who actually have appendicitis. What is this statistic called?

42. You investigate your test for appendicitis further and find that 74% of those who test negative for appendicitis are truly disease-free. What is this statistic called?

43. Your new test for appendicitis identifies 38% of patients who actually have appendicitis as being negative for appendicitis. What is this statistic called?

44. You are keen to determine whether smoking is a risk factor for a new disease that has been identified. You take the proportion of smokers who develop the disease and divide this by the proportion of non-smokers who develop the disease. What is this statistic called?

45. This new disease affects 28 new people per 100,000 per year. What is this statistic called?

Theme: macroscopic haematuria

Please answer each question with one of the following options. Each option may be used once, more than once or not at all.

a. Bladder stones

b. Renal stones

c. Bladder outlet obstruction

d. Prostatitis

e. Transitional cell carcinoma of the bladder

f. Renal cell carcinoma

g. Orchitis

h. Ureterocoele

i. Vesico-ureteric reflux

j. Pyocystitis

46. An 89-year-old male has visible haematuria, nocturia and poor stream. What is the most likely diagnosis?

47. A 65-year-old male smoker presents with visible haematuria. He has no other symptoms. What is the most likely diagnosis?

48. A 73-year-old male presents with visible haematuria and recurrent urinary tract infection (UTI). What is the most likely cause of his symptoms?

49. A 43-year-old female presents with visible haematuria and pain. She has an ileal conduit following a cystectomy for bladder cancer. What is the most likely cause of her symptoms?

50. A 23-year-old male presents with visible haematuria and perineal pain. What is the most likely cause of his symptoms?

MRCS Part A Paper 2

Mock Paper 8

Please answer all questions.

You have **45 minutes** to complete this paper.

Theme: thyroid disease

Please answer each question with one of the following options. Each option may be used once, more than once or not at all.

a. Graves' disease

b. Hashimoto's thyroiditis

c. Multinodular goitre

d. Anaplastic carcinoma

e. Medullary carcinoma

f. Follicular carcinoma

g. Follicular adenoma

h. Thyroid lymphoma

i. Thyroid lobectomy

j. Total thyroidectomy

1. A 35-year-old female presents with a diffuse goitre, feeling lethargic and sensitive to the cold. What is the most likely diagnosis?

2. A 35-year-old female presents with a diffuse goitre, palpitations and heat intolerance. What is the most likely diagnosis?

3. A 71-year-old male with a craggy anterior neck mass presents with weight loss and recent-onset hoarse voice. What is the most likely diagnosis?

4. What is the treatment of choice for a follicular adenoma?

5. What is the treatment of choice for a follicular carcinoma?

Theme: paediatric surgery

Please answer each question with one of the following options. Each option may be used once, more than once or not at all.

a. Constipation

b. Pyloric stenosis

c. Enterocolitis

d. Intussusception

e. Appendicitis

f. Gastroschisis

g. Gastroenteritis

h. Exomphalos

i. Mesenteric adenitis

j. Malrotation and volvulus

6. A 6-month-old male presents to the ED with intermittent colicky abdominal pain, during which he draws up his knees. His parents have noticed small amounts of blood in his nappy. An abdominal mass is palpable. What is the most likely pathology?

7. A 5-year-old female attends the ED with generalised abdominal pain. She has recently had an upper respiratory tract infection. She has a temperature of 38°C and has cervical lymphadenopathy. Her abdomen is mildly tender and the pattern of tenderness is variable. What is the most likely pathology?

8. A 6-week-old baby is brought to the ED with a 2-day history of projectile vomiting. Between vomiting episodes, he feeds well. A small mass is felt in the epigastrium during feeds. What is the most likely pathology?

9. A 15-year-old female presents with a 2-day history of generalised abdominal pain that has now localised to the right iliac fossa. She is vomiting and has a reduced appetite. On examination, you find there is guarding in the right iliac fossa and she has a temperature of 37.7°C. What is the most likely pathology?

10. A child is born with an abdominal wall defect to the right of the midline. The bowel is eviscerated through the defect, with no overlying sac. What is the most likely pathology?

Theme: abdominal imaging

Please answer each question with one of the following options. Each option may be used once, more than once or not at all.

a. CT scan of the abdomen/ pelvis

b. Colonoscopy

c. Mesenteric angiogram

d. Laparoscopy

e. Erect chest X-ray

f. Abdominal/pelvic USS

g. Laparotomy

h. Focused assessment with sonography for trauma scan

i. Abdominal X-ray

11. A 50-year-old female who takes diclofenac for osteoarthritis presents with severe epigastric pain. Her HR is 110 bpm and she is afebrile. What is the most appropriate *initial* investigation?

12. A 90-year-old female is brought to A&E with profuse dark red rectal bleeding. Despite vigorous resuscitation, her HR is 120 bpm and her BP is 80/50 mmHg. She has multiple co-morbidities, including a myocardial infarction that occurred 2 weeks ago. What is the most appropriate investigation?

13. A 2-year-old male presents with a 6-hour history of intermittent severe abdominal pain and vomiting. A mass is palpable in the right iliac fossa. He is not peritonitic. What is the most appropriate investigation?

14. A 40-year-old male attends clinic with a 3-month history of loose stools and intermittent rectal bleeding. The blood is mixed with the stool. Examination in clinic reveals no abnormalities. What is the most appropriate investigation?

15. An 80-year-old male is admitted with abdominal pain and distension. He has not opened his bowels for 3 days and has now started vomiting. On examination, you find his abdomen is tender but not peritonitic, and he is haemodynamically stable. What is the most appropriate *initial* investigation?

Theme: the acutely unwell surgical patient

Please answer each question with one of the following options. Each option may be used once, more than once or not at all.

a. Sepsis

b. Anaphylactic shock

c. Cardiogenic shock

d. Neurogenic shock

e. Hypovolaemic shock

f. Spinal shock

g. Pulmonary embolism

h. SIRS

i. Septic shock

j. Syncope

16. Twenty-four hours after a total hip replacement under spinal anaesthetic, a 50-year-old male becomes pale and sweaty. He has a HR of 120 bpm, a BP of 90/60 mmHg and a temperature of 37.2°C. His jugular venous pressure is raised and you can hear bibasal lung crackles. Which term best describes his clinical status?

17. Six hours after a small bowel resection, a 25-year-old female becomes confused. She has cool peripheries, a BP of 90/50 mmHg and a HR of 120 bpm. Her urine output has been 100 mL since leaving theatre. Which term best describes her clinical status?

18. An 8-month-old male has been lethargic and refusing to feed for 6 days. His HR is 160 bpm, RR is 50 breaths/min and temperature is 38.5°C. He has a positive urine dipstick. Which clinical term best describes his physiological status?

19. A 32-year-old alcoholic presents with epigastric pain that radiates to his back. His temperature is 38.0°C, HR is 100 bpm and BP is 125/85 mmHg. Which clinical term best describes his physiological status?

20. A 45-year-old female is undergoing wide local excision and sentinel node biopsy for breast cancer. Shortly following injection of the blue dye, the anaesthetist tells you he is having trouble maintaining her BP, which is now 60/40 mmHg. Her HR is 140 bpm. Which clinical term best describes her physiological status?

Theme: **Venous thromboembolism**

Please answer each question with one of the following options. Each option may be used once, more than once or not at all.

a. None

b. Compression pumps only

c. TED® stockings and LMWH

d. IV heparin infusion (therapeutic dose)

e. Warfarin

f. LMWH and compression pumps

g. TED® stockings only

h. LMWH only

21. A 35-year-old type 1 diabetic is admitted for an elective total knee replacement. He is a poorly controlled diabetic admitted for a preoperative insulin sliding scale. He has complications from his diabetes, including peripheral neuropathy. What VTE prophylaxis should he receive post-operatively?

22. A 55-year-old type 1 diabetic is admitted for an insulin sliding scale pre-elective left total hip replacement. He is due to have the operation done under spinal anaesthesia. He reports peripheral neuropathy and an ulcer on his right hallux. What VTE prophylaxis should he receive before his operation?

23. A 32-year-old female is admitted with acute appendicitis. She had a renal transplant for immunoglobulin A nephropathy 5 years ago. What VTE prophylaxis should she receive after her operation?

24. A 60-year-old male is readmitted following total hip replacement with a possible wound infection. What VTE prophylaxis should he receive?

25. A 75-year-old female is admitted with a fractured femoral neck. She has gross bilateral lymphoedema. What VTE prophylaxis should she receive after her operation?

Theme: **vascular disease**

Please answer each question with one of the following options. Each option may be used once, more than once or not at all.

a. Marjolin's ulcer

b. Chronic venous insufficiency

c. Deep vein thrombosis

d. Arterial disease

e. Lymphoedema

f. Cellulitis

g. Pyoderma gangrenosum

h. Four-layer compression bandages

i. No compression dressings

j. Amputation

26. A 65-year-old male has bilateral lipodermatosclerosis, haemosiderin deposition and 'inverted champagne bottle'-shaped legs. What is the diagnosis?

27. A 55-year-old female smoker has ulcerations over the gaiter region of her right leg. What is the most likely cause?

28. A 35-year-old air steward complains of aching and heaviness in her legs after long-haul flights. On examination, you find she has varicose veins along the course of the long saphenous vein. What must be excluded prior to definitive management?

29. A 60-year-old female develops an ulcer on the medial aspect of her right leg. Her ankle brachial pressure index (ABPI) is 1.1 on the left and 1.0 on the right. How would you manage her leg ulcer?

30. A 75-year-old female suffers from a chronic venous leg ulcer that fails to heal despite conservative treatment. Of what would you be suspicious?

Theme: ankle fractures

Please answer each question with one of the following options. Each option may be used once, more than once or not at all.

a. Closed reduction and cast

b. Antero-posterior (AP) and lateral plain films

c. AP, lateral and mortise plain films

d. AP, lateral and skyline plain films

e. CT scan of the ankle

f. Open reduction and internal fixation

g. Weber A

h. Weber B

i. Weber C

j. Maisonneuve fracture

k. Calcaneal fracture

31. A 35-year-old male sustains an ankle injury playing football. On examination, you find his ankle grossly swollen with obvious deformity of the joint. The foot is cold and you cannot feel pulses. After initial resuscitation according to the Advanced Trauma Life Support (ATLS) guidelines, what should you do next?

32. A 40-year-old female falls on an icy footpath and sustains a fracture of her distal fibula at the syndesmosis. What type of fracture is this?

33. How would you manage a Weber C fibula fracture?

34. A 50-year-old male sustains an ankle injury playing rugby. X-rays show a medial malleolus fracture and what looks like widening of the syndesmosis. What other fracture must you exclude?

35. When an ankle fracture is suspected, what imaging is initially required?

Theme: liver and biliary anatomy

Please answer each question with one of the following options. Each option may be used once, more than once or not at all.

a. Falciform ligament

b. Cardiac ligament

c. Quadrate lobe

d. Common bile duct

e. Cystic artery

f. Cystic duct

g. Mascagni's node

h. Epiploic foramen

i. Pringle's manoeuvre

j. Winslow's manoeuvre

36. You are performing a laparoscopic cholecystectomy and identify Calot's triangle. What structure forms its lateral border?

37. Other than the cystic artery, what is contained within Calot's triangle?

38. At laparotomy for a gunshot wound to the right upper quadrant, you try to gain control of bleeding from a liver laceration by compressing the hepatic artery and portal vein. What is this technique called?

39. Which ligament relating to the liver will be seen first during insertion of the epigastric port at laparoscopic cholecystectomy?

40. During a laparoscopic cholecystectomy, injury to which structure may lead to a bile leak?

Theme: pelvic injuries

Please answer each question with one of the following options. Each option may be used once, more than once or not at all.

a. Antero-posterior (AP) and lateral plain films

b. AP, lateral and swimmer's view plain films

c. AP, lateral and Judet view plain films

d. AP, lateral and mortise view plain films

e. Pubic ramus fracture

f. Acetabular fracture

g. Sciatic nerve

h. Obturator nerve

i. Femoral nerve

j. Anterior hip dislocation

k. Posterior hip dislocation

41. An 80-year-old female with a right total hip replacement complains of severe pain and inability to bear weight after trying to stand up from a low armchair. What is the most likely diagnosis?

42. A 35-year-old male is the front seat passenger in a road traffic accident. His left leg is shortened, internally rotated and held in adduction. What is the most likely diagnosis?

43. Which nerve must you formally assess in patients with an anterior hip dislocation?

44. An 85-year-old female has a fall. She describes pain over her right groin that is worse when bearing weight. What injury may she have sustained?

45. When suspecting a pelvic fracture, what imaging should you request?

Theme: flank pain

Please answer each question with one of the following options. Each option may be used once, more than once or not at all.

a. Renal colic

b. Ovarian torsion

c. Pyelonephritis

d. Renal cell carcinoma

e. Abdominal aortic aneurysm rupture

f. Thoracic aortic dissection

g. Diabetic ketoacidosis

h. Appendicitis

i. Pelvic inflammatory disease

j. Transitional cell bladder carcinoma

46. A 23-year-old female complains of right-sided flank pain with vomiting. Urine dipstick is positive for nitrites, protein and blood. She is pyrexial with a temperature of 38.4°C. What is the most likely diagnosis?

47. A 23-year-old male presents with left-sided abdominal pain and vomiting. He reports urinary frequency for several days. Urine dipstick is positive for glucose and ketones. He is apyrexial. What is the most likely diagnosis?

48. A 39-year-old male type 1 diabetic complains of severe left-sided flank pain and vomiting. He is requiring morphine. Urine dipstick is positive for blood. He is apyrexial. What is the most likely diagnosis?

49. A 65-year-old male smoker complains of severe left-sided abdominal pain. Urine dipstick is negative. He is apyrexial. His HR is 120 bpm and BP is 80/40 mmHg. What is the most likely diagnosis?

50. A 33-year-old male with a history of renal stones has right-sided abdominal pain in his lower abdomen that started centrally. Urine dipstick is negative. He is febrile with a temperature of 38.0°C. What is the most likely diagnosis?

MRCS Part A Paper 2

Mock Paper 9

Please answer all questions.

You have **45 minutes** to complete this paper.

Theme: neck lumps

Please answer each question with one of the following options. Each option may be used once, more than once or not at all.

a. Sebaceous cyst

b. Lipoma

c. Reactive lymph node

d. Thyroid nodule

e. Thyroglossal cyst

f. Cystic hygroma

g. Branchial cyst

h. Fibromatosis colli

i. Carotid body tumour

j. Malignant lymph node

1. A 10-year-old female complains of a painful lump in her neck, just below the mandible. She has recently had a sore throat and runny nose. On examination, you palpate several firm, mobile lumps in the cervical region. What is the most likely diagnosis?

2. A 45-year-old male is concerned about a lump on the back of his neck. It sometimes becomes red and tender. It feels attached to the skin. What is the most likely diagnosis?

3. A 15-year-old male presents with a midline neck lump. It moves upwards on swallowing or protrusion of the tongue. What is the most likely diagnosis?

4. A 2-year-old male presents with a swelling on the anterior border of the left sternocleidomastoid. What is the most likely diagnosis?

5. A 2-year-old female presents with a swelling in the left posterior triangle of the neck. She also has Turner's syndrome. What is the most likely diagnosis?

Theme: head injury

Please answer each question with one of the following options. Each option may be used once, more than once or not at all.

a. 0   g. 9

b. 1   h. 10

c. 3   i. 11

d. 4   j. 12

e. 5   k. 13

f. 6   l. 14

6. A 16-year-old with a head injury makes no verbal response to pain, is not opening his eyes to pain and makes no motor response to pain. What is his GCS score?

7. A 25-year-old with a head injury flexes his left arm in response to pain, opens his eyes to speech and is grunting. He withdraws his right arm from pain. What is his GCS score?

8. A 79-year-old female is talking but confused. She responds to pain by withdrawing and opens her eyes in response to pain. What is her GCS score?

9. A 50-year-old male has his eyes closed and extends his arms and moans in response to pain. What is his GCS score?

10. An 89-year-old female is following motor commands, has her eyes open and is talking but confused. What is her GCS score?

Theme: knee injuries

Please answer each question with one of the following options. Each option may be used once, more than once or not at all.

a. Diagnostic arthroscopy and washout

b. Diagnostic arthroscopy and/or meniscectomy

c. McMurray's test

d. Lachman's test

e. Posterior drawer test

f. Anterior cruciate ligament

g. Posterior cruciate ligament

h. Medial meniscal injury

i. Lateral meniscal injury

j. Lateral collateral ligament

k. Medial collateral ligament

l. X-ray

m. CT scan

11. A 45-year-old male sustains a knee injury while skiing. He reports there was twisting with his knee bent. Suddenly, his knee swelled and was exquisitely painful. What has he most likely injured?

12. What bedside test requires you to hold the patient's knee at 30 degrees of flexion, fixing the femur with one hand while using the other to apply anterior force to the calf, noting the degree of tibial displacement?

13. A 25-year-old female complains of medial knee pain. She plays sport regularly and reports that her knee swelled a few hours after playing netball last week. She has point tenderness over the medial joint line and is McMurray's-test positive. What is the most likely injury?

14. A 40-year-old male complains of knee pain and you suspect a medial meniscal injury. What other ligament must you also assess for injury?

15. A 30-year-old male has a suspected meniscal injury on MRI scan. What should you do next?

Theme: nutrition

Please answer each question with one of the following options. Each option may be used once, more than once or not at all.

a. Milkshake/juice supplements

b. Enteral feeding via NG tube

c. Parenteral feeding via central line

d. Parenteral feeding via femoral line

e. Enteral feeding via NJ tube

f. Oral intake

g. Line sepsis

h. Re-feeding syndrome

i. Systemic inflammatory response

16. A 75-year-old acute surgical patient has had minimal oral intake in the last 5 days. She has no appetite and is struggling to swallow food. What nutritional support could be considered?

17. A 35-year-old male with severe Crohn's disease has 120 cm of small bowel left after multiple previous resections. He has undergone an emergency laparotomy and adhesiolysis and is now day-2 post-operative. Which mode of nutritional support is most appropriate for him?

18. A 55-year-old patient with a perforated sigmoid diverticulum, faecal peritonitis and a defunctioning ileostomy has a high stoma output and has been on the intensive care unit (ICU) for 6 days, requiring respiratory support. Which route of nutritional support should be used for this patient?

19. A 65-year-old female with short gut syndrome is started on TPN before Easter bank holiday weekend. Her electrolytes are not checked and on Tuesday morning the nurses inform you she is confused and unable to get out of bed. Her observations are unremarkable. What could be causing her symptoms?

20. A 75-year-old male alcoholic is on the ward when he has a fall and sustains a neck-of-femur fracture. He becomes pyrexial following left hip hemiarthroplasty. He is being TPN fed due to a pancreatic pseudocyst. His wound looks clean and a full septic screen is undertaken with bloods from the central line, as he is difficult to bleed. What could be the cause of his symptoms?

Theme: shoulder injuries

Please answer each question with one of the following options. Each option may be used once, more than once or not at all.

a. Bankart lesion

b. Hill–Sachs lesion

c. Anterior dislocation

d. Posterior dislocation

e. Inferior dislocation

f. Axillary nerve function

g. Median nerve function

h. Brachial plexus

i. Lateral cutaneous nerve function

j. Rotator cuff injury

k. Humeral (surgical) neck fracture

21. While playing rugby, a 25-year-old male falls on an outstretched arm. He complains of pain in his shoulder and is unable to move the joint. On examination, you find fullness beneath the clavicle and that the normal contour of the shoulder has been lost. What injury might he have sustained?

22. An 18-year-old male is assaulted. He complains of severe pain in his shoulder and is unable to move his arm. His X-ray shows the 'light bulb' sign but no evidence of a fracture. What injury might this be?

23. A 40-year-old male suffers an anterior dislocation of his right shoulder after falling while ice skating. What must you assess before you attempt a closed reduction?

24. A 35-year-old female suffers anterior dislocation of her right shoulder with no neurovascular compromise. You successfully relocate the humeral head into the glenoid fossa. What must you assess next?

25. A 29-year-old male presents to A&E with a painful shoulder. He reports a history of recurrent dislocations and, on this occasion, the shoulder has spontaneously reduced. It hurts more than usual and is now clicking and popping as he moves. His X-ray shows a depression fracture of the posterior superior humeral head. What is this called?

Theme: ABG sampling

Please answer each question with one of the following options. Each option may be used once, more than once or not at all.

a. Large bowel obstruction

b. Gastric outlet obstruction

c. Anxiety

d. Diverticulitis

e. Peptic ulcer disease

f. Diabetic ketoacidosis

g. Hyperosmolar non-ketoacidosis

h. Pulmonary embolism

i. Ischaemic bowel

j. Appendicitis

26. A 68-year-old male smoker presents with vomiting. His ABG results are: pH 7.50; $PaCO_2$, 3.84; pO_2, 11.23; lactate, 1.9; K+, 2.8; Cl-, 80; HCO_3, 29; BE, +8.5; glucose, 5.3. What do these results imply the patient has?

27. An 85-year-old female in AF presents with generalised abdominal pain. Her ABG results are: pH 7.28; $PaCO_2$, 3.12; pO_2, 14.83; lactate, 5.7; K+, 4.8; Cl-, 98; HCO_3, 20; BE, –10.0; glucose, 4.8. What do these results imply the patient has?

28. A 50-year-old female with a new diagnosis of carcinoma of the left breast, presents feeling short of breath. Her ABG results are: pH 7.36; $PaCO_2$, 4.12; pO_2, 7.54; lactate, 1.2; K+, 3.9; Cl-, 101; HCO_3, 26; BE, –2.2; glucose, 5.4. What do these results imply the patient has?

29. A 25-year-old female presents to A&E with abdominal pain. Her RR is 30 breaths/min and she is complaining of circumoral tingling. Her ABG results are: pH 7.46; $PaCO_2$, 2.81; pO_2, 15.68; lactate, 1.1; K+, 4.0; Cl-, 100; HCO_3, 27; BE, +0.2; glucose, 4.7. What do these results imply the patient has?

30. A 37-year-old male presents 1 year after a pancreas transplant with abdominal pain and bloating. His ABG results are: pH 7.24; $PaCO_2$, 2.93; pO_2, 14.82; lactate, 2.0; K+, 6.8; Cl-, 99; HCO_3, 13; BE, –11.5; glucose, 20. What do these results imply the patient has?

Theme: autoimmune disease

Please answer each question with one of the following options. Each option may be used once, more than once or not at all.

a. Hashimoto's thyroiditis

b. Graves' disease

c. Atrophic gastritis

d. Pernicious anaemia

e. Myasthenia gravis

f. Goodpasture's syndrome

g. Systemic lupus erythematosus

h. Rheumatoid arthritis

i. Scleroderma

j. UC

31. Autoantibody screening detects anti-thyroglobulin antibodies in this disease.

32. Autoantibody screening detects antibodies to parietal cells in this disease.

33. Autoantibody screening detects antibodies to the glomerular basement membrane in this disease.

34. Autoantibody screening detects antibodies to acetylcholine receptors in this disease.

35. Autoantibody screening detects antibodies to centromere and anti-Scl-70 in this disease.

Theme: post-operative abdominal pain

Please answer each question with one of the following options. Each option may be used once, more than once or not at all.

a. Hypocalcaemia

b. Hypercalcaemia

c. Hyponatraemia

d. Hypernatraemia

e. Ileus

f. Upper GI bleed

g. Lower GI bleed

h. Anastomotic leak

i. Intra-abdominal collection

j. Retained foreign body

k. Abdominal compartment syndrome

36. A 67-year-old patient with metastatic renal cell carcinoma undergoes simple nephrectomy for disease debulking and symptom control of haematuria. He is complaining of generalised abdominal pain, constipation and general malaise. What is the most likely cause?

37. A 58-year-old patient is day-5 post radical cystectomy and neobladder formation for carcinoma in situ. He is complaining of lower abdominal pain. There is high output from his drain, which appears serous. His urine output has been 0 mL/h for the past 4 hours. What is the most likely post-operative complication causing these symptoms?

38. A 61-year-old patient is day-7 post anterior resection for rectal carcinoma. He is complaining of lower abdominal pain and has developed diarrhoea. His C-reactive protein (CRP) has been rising since the operation. What is the most likely pathology?

39. A 49-year-old patient is day-3 post repair of a perforated duodenal ulcer. He is complaining of abdominal discomfort and still has a high NG output. What is the most likely cause of this?

40. Eight hours after a delayed second-stage closure of laparostomy, performed due to gross faecal contamination following a perforated sigmoid diverticulum, a 38-year-old patient is tachycardic, hypertensive and complaining of severe abdominal pain. What is the most likely pathology responsible for his symptoms?

Theme: polypharmacy in the surgical patient

Please answer each question with one of the following options. Each option may be used once, more than once or not at all.

a. NSAID

b. Steroid

c. Cyclosporin

d. Tacrolimus

e. Mycophenolate

f. Gentamicin

g. Penicillin

h. Omeprazole

i. Rifampicin

j. Heparin

41. Which drug may cause sensorineural hearing loss?

42. Which drug may cause acne and fluid retention?

43. Which drug may cause jaundice and orange urine?

44. Which drug may cause a proximal myopathy?

45. Which drug may cause thrombocytopenia?

Theme: principles of surgical incisions

a. Lanz incision for appendectomy

b. Midline incision for laparotomy

c. Lumbar incision for nerve root decompression

d. Neck incision for tracheotomy

e. Neck incision for cricothyroidotomy

f. Lumbar puncture

g. Oblique incision for inguinal hernia repair

h. Midline raphe incision for testicular exploration

i. Incision for lateral approach to hip

j. Incision for carpal tunnel decompression

46. Which incision would you use to cut through the following layers: skin, subcutaneous tissue, tensor fasica lata, vastus medialis, vastus lateralis, gluteus medius, gluteus minimis and fibrous capsule?

47. Which incision would you use to cut through the following layers: skin, subcutaneous tissue (Camper's fascia), Scarpa's fascia and external oblique?

48. Which incision would you use to cut through the following layers: skin, subcutaneous tissue, dartos muscle and tunica vaginalis?

49. Which incision would you use to cut through the following layers: skin, subcutaneous tissue, deep fascia, supraspinous ligament, interspinous ligament, ligamentum flavum, dura mater and arachnoid mater?

50. Which incision would you use to cut through the following layers: skin, subcutaneous tissue and flexor retinaculum?

MRCS Part A Paper 2

Mock Paper 10

Please answer all questions.

You have **45 minutes** to complete this paper.

Theme: breast disease

Please answer each question with one of the following options. Each option may be used once, more than once or not at all.

a. USS and FNA

b. Mammography and FNA

c. Reassurance

d. DCIS

e. Carcinoma

f. Fibroadenoma

g. Fat necrosis

h. Mastectomy

i. Wide local excision

1. A 20-year-old female who is otherwise fit and well presents with a small, mobile breast lump. What is the most likely diagnosis?

2. A 67-year-old female presents with a hard craggy mass in her right breast. What is the most appropriate investigation/management?

3. A slim 61-year-old female has a 5 cm invasive ductal carcinoma of the left breast. What is the most appropriate surgical management in this case?

4. An 18-year-old female presents to her general practitioner with bilateral cyclical breast pain. Clinical examination is unremarkable. What is the most appropriate investigation/management?

5. A 31-year-old female presents with a smooth cystic lesion in her left breast. What is the most appropriate investigation/management?

Theme: proximal femur fractures

Please answer each question with one of the following options. Each option may be used once, more than once or not at all.

a. Assess fitness for surgery

b. Assess 'do not attempt resuscitation' status

c. Dynamic hip screw

d. Cannulated screws

e. Cemented hip hemiarthroplasty

f. Uncemented hemiarthroplasty

g. Total hip replacement

h. Proximal femoral nail

i. Neurovascular status of the limb

6. An 80-year-old female falls out of bed. She sustains a subcapital, undisplaced, impacted (Garden stage I) right neck-of-femur fracture. How would you fix this?

7. An 85-year-old male falls at home. He sustains a right subtrochanteric neck-of-femur fracture. How would you fix this?

8. While out shopping, a 75-year-old female falls. She sustains a left intertrochanteric neck-of-femur fracture. How would you fix this?

9. An 87-year-old male falls at home. On examination, you find his right leg is shortened and externally rotated. In this situation, what must you always assess as part of your initial clinical examination?

10. A 70-year-old female with osteoporosis, type 2 diabetes mellitus and AF has an undisplaced left neck-of-femur fracture. Distal neurovascular status is intact. What must you first assess before a definitive management decision can be made?

Theme: systemic inflammatory response

Please answer each question with one of the following options. Each option may be used once, more than once or not at all.

a. Soft tissue infection

b. Infected prosthesis

c. Reperfusion injury

d. Major haemorrhage

e. Rhabdomyolysis

f. Lactate >1.2 mmol/L

g. PaO_2 <9.3 kPa

h. Urine output <120 mL over 4 hours

i. GCS score <15 in absence of sedation/central nervous system (CNS) lesion

j. Refractory hypotension

11. A 50-year-old patient is found with a temperature of 38.5°C, a white cell count (WCC) of 16.3 × 10^9/L and is confused and distressed 3 days after a right open reduction internal fixation of a compound tibia and fibula. The operative wound is erythematous with some sloughy ooze. What is the cause of her SIRS?

12. A 75-year-old male undergoes left femoral embolectomy for an acutely ischaemic limb. Six hours after the operation, on the ward his HR is 105 bpm, RR is 24 breaths/min and he is mildly confused. His potassium is 6.2 mmol/L on venous gas. What is the cause of his SIRS?

13. A 65-year-old male with a diabetic foot and wet gangrene of his great hallux is unwell. His temperature is 39.5°C, HR is 125 bpm and blood sugars are erratic, even on an insulin sliding scale. What is the biochemical definition of cardiovascular system compromise?

14. A 55-year-old female diabetic suffers chronic osteomyelitis of her right hallux. She is admitted with an acutely swollen right leg with marked erythema. Her temperature is 38.2°C, HR is 100 bpm and WCC is 32 × 10^9/L. What is the cause of her SIRS?

15. A 70-year-old male has confirmed staphylococcal sepsis of his right hip hemiarthroplasty. He is unstable, with a BP of 85/40 mmHg, HR of 120 bpm and O_2 saturations of 90% on room air. In the presence of an identified infective organism what else do you require to classify a patient as suffering from 'septic shock'?

Theme: forearm fractures

Please answer each question with one of the following options. Each option may be used once, more than once or not at all.

a. Greenstick fracture

b. Antibiotic cover

c. Tetanus status

d. Monteggia fracture

e. Osteoarthritis

f. Malunion

g. Non-union

h. Galeazzi fracture

i. Complex regional pain syndrome

j. Osteoporosis

16. A 55-year-old male falls and his X-ray shows a fracture of the ulnar shaft with dislocation of the radial head. What fracture is this?

17. A 40-year-old male falls and X-ray shows a fracture of the distal radial shaft with dislocation of the radioulnar joint. What is this fracture called?

18. A 60-year-old male has a nasty fall in his allotment, sustaining an open forearm fracture. You wash the wound with saline and cover it with a povidone iodine-soaked gauze. In this situation, what should you assess when taking the patient's history?

19. A 32-year-old female falls from her bicycle and lands on her out-stretched hand. She sustains a distal radius fracture of her dominant hand with volar angulation. The fracture extends into the joint line and there appears to be displacement of the carpus bones. What long-term complication should you inform the patient she is at increased risk of?

20. A 45-year-old female undergoes elective carpal tunnel decompression. What long-term complication should you warn her of when obtaining her consent for the procedure?

Theme: principles of surgical incisions

Please answer each question with one of the following options. Each option may be used once, more than once or not at all.

a. Lanz incision for appendectomy

b. Midline incision for laparotomy

c. Lumbar incision for nerve root decompression

d. Neck incision for tracheotomy

e. Incision for carpal tunnel decompression

f. Lumbar puncture

g. Oblique incision for inguinal hernia repair

h. Midline raphe incision for testicular exploration

i. Incision for lateral approach to hip

j. Neck incision for cricothyroidotomy

21. Which incision would you use to cut through skin, subcutaneous tissue, the linea alba and the peritoneum?

22. Which incision would you use to cut through skin, subcutaneous tissue, the platysma, the investing layer of the deep cervical fascia, strap muscles, the pre-tracheal fascia, the thyroid isthmus and the trachea?

23. Which incision would you use to cut through skin, subcutaneous tissue, platysma, the investing layer of the deep cervical fascia, strap muscles, the pre-tracheal fascia and the cricothyroid membrane?

24. Which incision would you use to cut through skin, subcutaneous tissue (Camper's fascia), Scarpa's fascia, the external oblique, the internal oblique, the transversus abdominis, the transversalis fascia, pre-peritoneal fat and the peritoneum?

25. Which incision would you use to cut through skin, subcutaneous tissue, deep fascia, the supraspinous ligament, the interspinous ligament and ligamentum flavum?

Theme: the red eye

Please answer each question with one of the following options. Each option may be used once, more than once or not at all.

a. Conjunctivitis

b. Lagophthalmos

c. Subconjunctival haemorrhage

d. Dacryocystitis

e. Keratitis

f. Acute angle glaucoma

g. Episcleritis

h. Blepharitis

i. Trichiasis

j. Canaliculitis

26. A 7-year-old female presents with itchy and red eyes. On examination, you notice a discharge from both eyes. What is the most likely diagnosis?

27. A 60-year-old patient has noticed a small red patch on her right eye. It is not painful and she denies any other symptoms. On inspection, you find there is a small red area on the eyeball but nothing else of note. What is the most likely diagnosis?

28. A 35-year-old male complains of the sensation of a foreign body in his eye. He wears contact lenses but is confident he removed them. On inspection, you observe no obvious foreign body, but you see a corneal defect. What is the most likely diagnosis?

29. A 50-year-old male complains of a headache and severe left eye pain. He is photophobic and says his left eye will not stop watering. On inspection, you note that his left pupil is mid-dilated and fixed. What is the most likely diagnosis?

30. A 75-year-old male presents with a very bloody eye following a week-long coryzal illness in which he was coughing a great deal. What is the most likely diagnosis?

Theme: heart valve disease

Please answer each question with one of the following options. Each option may be used once, more than once or not at all.

a. Aortic stenosis

b. Mitral stenosis

c. Aortic regurgitation

d. Pulmonary stenosis

e. Mitral regurgitation

f. Rheumatic fever

g. Congenital bicuspid valve

h. Flow murmur

i. Collapsing pulse

j. Narrow pulse pressure

31. A 45-year-old male is diagnosed with aortic stenosis. He is otherwise fit and well with no previous medical history. What is the most likely cause of his valvular disease?

32. Which clinical sign is evidence of aortic stenosis?

33. A patient has a diastolic murmur that radiates to the carotids. On examination, which clinical sign are you most likely to find?

34. A 32-year-old female who is 34-weeks pregnant and otherwise fit and well with no previous medical history has an incidental murmur heard on routine prenatal examination. What is the most likely diagnosis?

35. A 47-year-old male has a pansystolic murmur that radiates to his apex, which is displaced laterally and inferiorly. What is the most likely diagnosis?

Theme: surgical infections

Please answer each question with one of the following options. Each option may be used once, more than once or not at all.

a. *Cytomegalovirus*

b. *Streptococcus pneumoniae*

c. Human immunodeficiency virus (HIV)

d. *Mycoplasma tuberculosis*

e. *Pseudomonas aeruginosa*

f. *Streptococcus pyogenes*

g. *Staphylococcus aureus*

h. Human papillomavirus

i. *Staphylococcus epidermidis*

j. *Bacteroides fragilis*

36. A 40-year-old male is admitted with diarrhoea, myalgia and malaise a month after receiving a kidney transplant. His temperature is 37.6°C. His recent blood tests show his immunosuppression levels are high. What organism is most likely to be causing these symptoms?

37. A 60-year-old female presents with hip pain 3 weeks after a hip replacement. Further investigation shows that the pathogen is a Gram-positive coccus that forms clusters and produces slime. What organism is most likely to be causing her symptoms?

38. A 70-year-old female attends clinic with a leg ulcer that will not heal. The skin around the ulcer is erythematic and there is a greenish exudate from the wound. What organism is most likely to be responsible?

39. A 30-year-old male is admitted 2 years post splenectomy with pyrexia and rigors. On examination, you find he has course crepitations in both lung bases. What organism is most likely to be causing his symptoms?

40. A 45-year-old male with type 1 diabetes mellitus presents to the ED with an extremely painful, erythematic leg following an insect bite. The erythema is spreading rapidly and he is febrile and tachycardic. Blood cultures are sent and a Gram-positive coccus is identified that occurs in chains. It is a facultative anaerobe. What organism is most likely to be making the patient ill?

Theme: abdominal pain

Please answer each question with one of the following options. Each option may be used once, more than once or not at all.

a. Duodenal ulcer

b. Gastric ulcer

c. Biliary colic

d. Ruptured aortic aneurysm

e. Acute cholecystitis

f. Ascending cholangitis

g. Diverticulitis

h. UTI

i. Perforated viscus

j. Ureteric colic

41. A 32-year-old female attends clinic complaining of a 3-month history of intermittent abdominal pain an hour after meals. She thinks it is worse when she eats cheese. Today she started vomiting during a painful episode and has a temperature of 38°C. What is the most likely diagnosis?

42. A 30-year-old male develops severe pain in his loin that radiates to the groin. He is restless and unable to find a comfortable position. On urinalysis, there is non-visible haematuria. What is the most likely diagnosis?

43. A 70-year-old female attends the ED with left iliac fossa pain and nausea. She is opening her bowels but reports some recent constipation. On examination, you find she is very tender in the left iliac fossa but her abdomen is otherwise soft. She is febrile. What is the most likely diagnosis?

44. A 65-year-old male complains of sudden-onset central abdominal pain that came on today. He has a history of ischaemic heart disease and has had a TIA. His BP on arrival at hospital is 60/40mmHg. What is the most likely diagnosis?

45. A 40-year-old female attends clinic with a 2-month history of epigastric pain. Eating relieves it. She also complains of bloating and often belches following a meal. She recently completed a course of steroids for an asthma exacerbation. What is the most likely diagnosis?

Theme: consent

Please answer each question with one of the following options. Each option may be used once, more than once or not at all.

a. Consent Form 1

b. Consent Form 2

c. Consent Form 3

d. Consent Form 4

e. Verbal consent

f. No consent required

g. Advanced directive

h. Power of attorney

i. Gillick competent/meets criteria of Fraser Guidelines

j. Ward of the court

46. A 23-year-old female involved in a road traffic accident sustains a severe head injury and arrives intubated and ventilated. She develops a tension pneumothorax that you wish to treat urgently. What kind of consent, if any, should be sought before the patient is treated?

47. An 18-year-old male with suspected appendicitis requires an operation. What kind of consent, if any, should be sought before the patient is treated?

48. A 10-year-old male with suspected testicular torsion requires an operation. What kind of consent, if any, should be sought before the patient is treated?

49. A 78-year-old female with vascular dementia and an abbreviated mental test score (AMTS) of 3 has an acute abdomen requiring an operation. What kind of consent, if any, should be sought before the patient is treated?

50. An 80-year-old male with an AMTS of 10 requires a closed reduction and backslab application to a fractured distal radius. What kind of consent, if any, should be sought before the patient is treated?

MRCS Part A Paper 1

Mock Paper 1

ANSWERS

1. **Masseter muscle.** The following are derived from the first branchial arch:
   - bones: malleus and incus of the middle ear, maxilla and mandible, palatine bone, the squamous part of the temporal bone and the spine of the sphenoid bone
   - muscles: masseter, the two pterygoids, temporalis, mylohyoid, anterior belly of digastric, tensor palati and tensor tympani
   - the mucous membrane and glands of the anterior two-thirds of the tongue.

   The hyoid bone derives from the second (lesser cornu and superior body) and third (greater cornu and inferior body) branchial arches. The posterior belly of the digastric muscle derives from the second branchial arch.

2. **All of the above.** The middle mediastinum contains the heart and pericardium, ascending aorta, superior vena cava (with the azygous vein opening into it), the bifurcation of the trachea and two main bronchi, the pulmonary artery, right and left pulmonary veins and the phrenic nerves. It does not contain the inferior vena cava.

3. **Right internal iliac artery.** 'Claudication' is muscular pain secondary to hypoxia. The buttocks are made up of three gluteal muscles: the piriformis, the gemellus (superior and inferior) and obturator

internus. They are mostly supplied by the superior and inferior gluteal arteries, both branches of the internal iliac artery.

4. **Varicose veins.** Varicose veins are not a recognised risk factor for VTE.

5. **Papillary carcinoma.** Papillary thyroid carcinoma accounts for 75%–85% of cases, follicular for 10%–20% of cases, medullary for 5%–8% of cases and anaplastic and thyroid lymphoma for <5%.

6. **Ilioinguinal nerve.** The ilioinguinal nerve is often exposed during an inguinal hernia repair. It supplies sensation to the medial thigh and anterior scrotum. Patients should be informed of the risk for damage to the nerve during the procedure.

7. **Superior epigastric artery.** Blood is supplied to the breast from three sources: the internal thoracic artery, the axillary artery (predominantly via the lateral thoracic and acromiothoracic branches) and the intercostal arteries.

8. **Coeliac trunk – T12/L1.** The main branches of the abdominal aorta are shown in the following table.

Single branches	
Coeliac	T12/L1
Superior mesenteric	L1
Inferior mesenteric	L3
Median sacral	L4
Paired branches	
Inferior phrenic	T12
Suprarenal	L1
Renal	L1/L2
Gonadal	L2
Lumbar (four pairs)	L1–4

9. **Sodium <130 mmol/L.** The need for renal replacement therapy will depend on the individual patient and their current medical status and medical history. However, for most patients, renal replacement therapy should be considered for: hyperkalaemia (persistently

>6 mmol/L), metabolic acidosis (pH <7.2), fluid overload/pulmonary oedema, urea >30 mmol/L, rapidly rising creatinine (>100 mmol/L/day), uraemia with complications (e.g. encephalopathy) and to aid drug clearance.

10. **Hypercitraturia.** The other answers are factors increasing the risk of formation of renal calculi.

11. **Anterior dislocation of the shoulder.** Falling on an outstretched arm is a common way a shoulder dislocation is sustained. Posterior dislocations are less common, occurring following epileptic fits, violent assaults or electric shocks. In anterior dislocation, which is more common, the humeral head sits on the anterior chest wall beneath the clavicle and results in the arm being internally rotated and held in adduction.

12. **Iliac crests.** The bony landmarks for a lumbar puncture are the iliac crests. The supracrestal plane intersects the vertebral column at L4, and the needle should be ideally inserted at L4/5.

13. **Pulmonary embolus.** Orthopaedic surgery and long periods of immobility are risk factors for thromboembolic disease. In this case, the patient shows clinical signs of hypoxia, tachypnoea and tachycardia consistent with a pulmonary embolus.

14. **Epidural.** Epidurals contain local anaesthetic with or without opioids. Their effect can mimic neurogenic shock by causing sympathetic blockade, leading to vasodilatation and hypotension. If the block is high enough or migrates while the patient is supine, bradycardia from unopposed parasympathetic action on the heart can ensue. The result will be reduced renal perfusion pressure, demonstrated by this patient's oliguria. All other options in this question should cause a tachycardia.

15. **6–8 weeks.** Recovery from neurapraxia is fast and a full recovery is usually made. On average, a neurapraxia will take 6–8 weeks to recover, although recovery time can range from days to months.

16. **Osteosarcoma.** Osteosarcoma is associated with a defect in the Rb1 gene, which also causes retinoblastoma.

17. **Age-related sclerosis.** Age-related sclerosis accounts for >50% of cases of aortic stenosis in the United Kingdom. A congenitally

bicuspid valve accounts for 30%–40% of cases. Marfan's syndrome and infective endocarditis will cause aortic regurgitation rather than stenosis. Rheumatic fever also causes aortic stenosis but is rare in the developed world.

18. **TNF-alpha is important for granuloma wall integrity.** Monoclonal antibodies that inhibit TNF-alpha, such as infliximab, may cause reactivation of latent TB due to breakdown of the granuloma wall. The stain of choice is Ziehl–Neelsen. Transmission may occur via droplet inhalation, ingestion of infected food and transplacentally but not through breast milk. When infectious, mothers are advised against close contact with their infants (including breastfeeding) due to droplet spread. The lung is the most common site of primary TB infection, but the pharynx, larynx, skin and intestine are also primary sites.

19. **Frank–Starling law.** Laplace's law describes the capillary pressure difference between two different fluids (e.g. air and blood in the lung). Poiseuille's law dictates that the flow through a tube is inversely proportional to the tube's radius to the power of four. Fick's law dictates that the rate of O_2 consumption is proportional to blood flow. Courvoisier's law states that painless jaundice with a palpable gallbladder is unlikely to be due to gallstones.

20. **Osteomalacia.** Osteomalacia is typified by soft bone due to reduced bone mineralisation.

21. **Parathyroid adenoma.** Parathyroid adenoma is a cause of primary hyperparathyroidism, generating hypercalcaemia and high serum PTH levels. The other answer options are all causes of secondary hyperparathyroidism, characterised by raised serum PTH levels with normal or reduced serum calcium levels.

22. **Oxytocin.** Oxytocin and vasopressin (antidiuretic hormone [ADH]) are the only hormones secreted by the posterior pituitary. The others are secreted by the anterior pituitary.

23. **PGE2 – dolor (pain).** The Greek scholar Celsus described the five cardinal signs of acute inflammation: rubor (redness), calor (heat), functio laesa (loss of function), tumour (swelling) and dolor (pain). Prostaglandins and nitric oxide cause vasodilation, leading to rubor

and calor. The complement cascade, leukotrienes, serotonin and histamine increase vascular permeability, leading to oedema, tumour and functio laesa. Dolor is caused by degranulation of lysosomes within the cell, releasing hyperalgesic chemical mediators such as PGE2.

24. **Budesonide.** Steroids are a recognised cause of pancreatitis.

25. **Chromosome replication occurs in S phase.** The cell cycle has five discrete phases. 'M phase' refers to cell division/mitosis. The G_1 and G_2 phases are pre-synthetic and pre-mitotic, respectively, but cells are not quiescent, as they are preparing for the next growth phase.

26. **Li–Fraumeni – p53 gene.** The MET gene is associated with papillary renal cell carcinoma. The Rb1 gene is associated with retinoblastoma, the RET gene is associated with MEN 2, the BRCA 1 and 2 genes are associated with prostate cancer and the NF1 gene is associated with NF. The APC gene is associated with FAP, whereas HNPCC is attributed to the MLH1, MSH 2 and 3 and PMS 1 and 2 genes.

27. **Middle meningeal artery**

28. **Mandibular.** The temporal and zygomatic are branches of the facial nerve.

29. **Arch of aorta.** When supine, the line drawn through the angle of Louis (T4/5) passes through the bifurcation of the trachea and the arch of the aorta lies just superior. On standing, gravity shifts everything downwards. The left venous angle is the junction of the left subclavian vein and internal jugular vein, which sits behind the left sternoclavicular joint. The left recurrent laryngeal nerve hooks under the arch of the aorta before ascending, whereas the right hooks under the right subclavian artery.

30. **The median nerve is derived from branches of the medial and lateral cords.** It helps to practise drawing the brachial plexus. The long thoracic nerve derives from C5, 6 and 7. The cords are named in relation to the second part of the axillary artery. The median cutaneous nerve of the forearm branches off the medial cord and is sensory. The musculocutaneous nerve supplies the biceps brachii, brachialis and coracobrachialis. It terminates as the lateral cutaneous nerve of the forearm, which is sensory.

31. **Ovaries.** All other structures are retroperitoneal, including the second, third and fourth parts of the duodenum and the pancreas (except the tail). The ovaries and uterus are intra-peritoneal.

32. **Popliteal artery.** The contents of the popliteal fossa, from deep to superficial, are the popliteal artery, popliteal vein and tibial nerve. The short saphenous vein lies in the subcutaneous tissue.

33. **Microangiopathic changes result in impaired wound healing.** Smoking increases HR and O_2 demand. O_2-carrying capacity is reduced by carboxyhaemoglobin, which binds haemoglobin, so less O_2 is offloaded to tissues – that is, the O_2–haemoglobin dissociation curve shifts to the left. Interestingly, stopping smoking even 24 hours before surgery will improve cardiovascular function, but patients are more likely to cough, which may affect hernia recurrence rates.

34. **The coagulation mode uses short bursts of high-voltage energy to desiccate tissue.** Accidental burns often happen through coupling. Direct coupling requires direct contact, whereas capacitance coupling involves the build-up of charge within a capacitor (in this case, air in the abdomen), which is then discharged at random. Hybrid ports (metal and plastic) increase the risk of this. Patients must not be in contact with a grounded metal object other than the diathermy plate itself. A pacemaker is a relative contraindication to monopolar diathermy. The cutting mode uses low-voltage continuous energy to produce high temperatures and vaporise tissues.

35. **The epidural could cause post-operative hypotension.** Epidurals usually contain a mixture of an opiate and local anaesthetic, although they can comprise just one agent. Ideally, an epidural should just cause sensory blockade but may be a cause of hypotension when peripheral vascular tone is affected. Asthma is not a contraindication to an epidural. Bupivacaine blocks voltage-gated sodium channels. NSAIDs inhibit COX and, therefore, prostaglandin formation.

36. **Cephalosporins.** Approximately 5%–10% of patients with a true penicillin allergy will be sensitive to cephalosporins (due to cross-reactivity), so they should be used with care.

37. **Aspiration is a common complication of enteral feeding.** The preferred method of feeding is enteral (i.e. via the gut), when it is safe.

Parenteral feeding (via a central line) is used when enteral feeding cannot be started. Marked interstitial fluid retention is seen as part of the metabolic response to sepsis and SIRS.

38. **Alkalosis shifts the O_2–haemoglobin dissociation curve to the left.** This increases haemoglobin's affinity for O_2. Hypoventilation occurs in respiratory compensation (raising the $PaCO_2$) but consequently lowers pO_2.

39. **>30 mmHg.** Fasciotomy is usually advocated for pressures >30 mmHg. Alternatively, you can be guided by the difference between compartment pressures and diastolic BP. Normal compartment pressures are 0–10 mmHg. In reality, they are not usually formally measured, as diagnosis is based on clinical findings.

40. **30–40 mL/kg/day.** The average adult requires 2–3 L of fluid per day, a large proportion of which comes from the food we eat.

41. **BPAP.** This woman has type II respiratory failure (hypoxic and hypercarbic). In the first instance, non-invasive ventilatory support should be considered. CPAP is required for type I respiratory failure (hypoxia only). BPAP is required for type II respiratory failure. When giving O_2, be mindful of COPD patients who may rely on a hypoxic drive to breathe.

42. **Smoking.** Smoking is a recognised risk factor for gastric cancer, along with male sex, an affected first-degree relative, eating spicy foods, pernicious anaemia, stomach lymphoma and *Helicobacter pylori* infection. Barrett's oesophagus is a risk factor for oesophageal adenocarcinoma.

43. **Fibroadenoma.** This is the typical history of a fibroadenoma, which is the most common abnormality in this age group.

44. **Metabolic acidosis with respiratory compensation.** The primary acid–base disturbance will be a metabolic acidosis due to ketosis. However, his RR of 30 breaths/min shows that he is compensating by attempting to blow off CO_2 in order to raise his pH.

45. **All of the above.** All these factors shift the O_2–haemoglobin curve to the left.

46. **4 hours.** For elective anaesthesia, infants are allowed formula milk or other solids up to 6 hours before their operation; breast milk until 4 hours before and clear fluids until 2 hours before, the same as for

adults. In an emergency, the fasting rules are the same (to reduce aspiration risk); however, the benefit of waiting for a child to be fasted must be weighed up against the risk of delaying surgery and, if necessary, a rapid sequence induction of anaesthesia may be performed if the operation cannot wait until the child is fasted.

47. **8.** The GCS score is determined from a patient's best response – in this case, his right arm localising pain (as opposed to his left arm extending from pain).

48. **Evisceration of bowel.** DPL is absolutely contraindicated in situations in which the patient needs an urgent laparotomy anyway (that is DPL will not change your subsequent management).

49. **4000 mL.** Burns resuscitation is dictated by the Parkland formula: 4 mL × body weight (kg) × total body surface area burned (%) for the first 24 hours, with 50% of this volume given in the first 8 hours and 50% in the subsequent 16 hours.

50. **Right optic tract.** This kind of visual field defect is called a 'homonymous hemianopia'. It occurs due to damage to the optic tract, or due to extensive damage to the optic radiation. Damage to only one part of the optic radiation may cause a homonymous quadrantanopia. Fibres have already crossed in the optic chiasm by this point, so the lesion affects both eyes, and a lesion on one side causes a visual field defect on the other. Compression of the optic chiasm would cause a bi-temporal hemianopia. An optic nerve lesion would affect one eye only.

MRCS Part A Paper 1

Mock Paper 2

ANSWERS

1. **T12 – azygos vein.** T8 is the caval opening, carrying the inferior vena cava and branches of the right phrenic nerve. T10 is the oesophageal hiatus, carrying the oesophagus, anterior and posterior vagal trunks. T12, the aortic hiatus, carries the aorta, azygous vein and thoracic duct.

2. **Prolactinoma.** MEN 1 (or Wermer's syndrome) is associated with pancreatic islet cell tumours, pituitary tumours (most commonly, prolactinomata) and parathyroid adenomata. MEN 2 is associated with phaeochromocytoma and medullary thyroid carcinoma with either parathyroid hyperplasia/tumour (MEN 2A) or mucocutaneous fibromata (MEN 2B).

3. **Superior mesenteric artery.** The coeliac artery supplies the foregut (from the mouth to the second part of the duodenum). The superior mesenteric artery supplies the midgut (from the second part of the duodenum to two-thirds of the way along the transverse colon). The inferior mesenteric artery supplies the hindgut. The lower left colic artery is a branch of the inferior mesenteric. The superior epigastric artery supplies the rectus abdominis.

4. **All of the above.** The spermatic cord contains three arteries (the testicular artery, cremasteric artery and artery to the vas deferens), two nerves (the genital branch of the genitofemoral nerve and sympathetic nerves), lymphatics, the pampiniform plexus and the vas deferens.

Note that the ilioinguinal nerve does not run within the spermatic cord.

5. **Sinus tachycardia.** The classic ECG changes associated with a pulmonary embolus are S1, Q3, T3 (a prominent S wave in lead 1, and a Q wave and inverted T wave in lead 3). However, the majority of patients with a pulmonary embolism will not display these changes. A sinus tachycardia is a very common finding in these patients.

6. **Inflammation confined to the mucosal and submucosal layers of the bowel wall.** The other answer options are more suggestive of Crohn's disease. UC is an inflammatory disease affecting the mucosa and submucosa of the bowel wall. UC extends proximally from the rectum for a variable distance around the colon. There are no skip lesions. Crohn's disease affects the full thickness of the bowel wall and is characterised by the presence of non-caseating granulomata. It can affect any part of the bowel, from mouth to anus, and there may be gaps between areas of inflammation. Anal Crohn's can lead to the presence of complex perianal fistulas, which can be problematic to treat. At operation, fatty encroachment of the serosa may be noted in Crohn's but not in UC.

7. **Axillary nerve.** This nerve provides sensory supply to the skin overlying the lateral aspect of the deltoid. Therefore, it is described as the 'regimental patch area', which refers to where patches are sited on military uniforms. It should be tested before and after dislocated shoulder joint reductions to ensure that there is no neurological damage. If there is abnormal neurology, surgical exploration is indicated.

8. **Opiate overdose.** Opiates cause respiratory depression and drowsiness. In fact, drowsiness is an early sign of impending opiate overdose.

9. **Granulation tissue formation.** Healing by primary intention involves wound-edge approximation, usually with sutures, to aid and promote faster wound healing. In healing by secondary intention, the wound edges are left apart and granulation tissue forms, with eventual epithelialisation, which is much slower. A VAC dressing can be used on some wounds that are healing by secondary intention to increase the rate of healing. Tertiary closure (delayed primary closure) can be a straightforward skin closure, or use tissue grafts to cover the wound.

10. **Takayasu's arteritis.** Takayasu's arteritis affects large vessels, typically the aorta and brachiocephalic trunks. Polyarteritis nodosa, Churg–Strauss and Wegener's granulomatosis affect medium- and small-sized arteries. Henoch–Schönlein purpura affects small vessels.

11. **Haemophilia B.** Haemophilia B is hereditary factor IX deficiency. Haemophilia A is hereditary factor VIII deficiency and von Willebrand's disease is hereditary von Willebrand factor deficiency. Glanzmann's disease and Bernard–Soulier syndrome are both hereditary platelet disorders.

12. **Acoustic neuromas are seen in NF2.** NF is inherited in an autosomal dominant pattern. Café au lait spots are due to melanocyte dysfunction in NF1. Acoustic neuromas may be seen in NF2. Schwannomas are associated with NF2. There are five recognised forms of NF.

13. **Bouchard's nodes.** Pannus, swan neck deformities and Boutonniere's deformities are typical of rheumatoid arthritis. Bouchard's (in the proximal interphalangeal [PIP] joints) and Heberden's (in the distal interphalangeal [DIP] joints) nodes are associated with osteoarthritis. Tophi are associated with gout.

14. **Meigs' syndrome.** Meigs' syndrome is a triad of ascites, transudative pleural effusion and benign ovarian tumour.

15. **Ventricular septal defect.** Non-cyanotic congenital heart disease occurs in a left-to-right shunt, so blood continues to travel to the lungs. A right-to-left shunt will cause cyanotic congenital cardiac disease, as the blood bypasses the lungs. Eisenmenger's syndrome is a left-to-right shunt that is then reversed due to pulmonary hypertension.

16. **Sino-atrial node.** The sino-atrial node has an intrinsic firing rate of 60–100 bpm. Other parts of the heart have a slower intrinsic firing rate.

17. **Adrenal cortical adenoma.** An adrenal cortical adenoma causes primary hyperaldosteronism, causing increased renal sodium reabsorption and potassium loss. Secondary hyperaldosteronism is caused by increased angiotensin II production and is associated with increased renin levels. Causes include heart failure, cirrhosis and

nephrotic syndrome. Phaeochromocytoma is an adrenal tumour that causes hypertension via increased catecholamine release, rather than affecting the renin–angiotensin system.

18. **The teres minor inserts into the most inferior part of the greater tubercle of the humerus.** Supraspinatus, infraspinatus and teres minor insert into the greater tubercle of the humerus (superior to inferior, respectively). The subscapularis inserts into the lesser tubercle of the humerus.

19. **C5a is chemotactic.** Neutrophils are the predominant cell type in the first 24 hours following injury; macrophages are involved after 48 hours. Prostaglandins and nitric oxide release cause smooth muscle relaxation. C3a, along with C5a, increases vascular permeability. C3b initiates the lytic pathway that produces the membrane attack complex.

20. **Interphase.** Chromosomes are replicated in interphase, then centrioles move to each pole of the cell and spindles form in prophase. Following this, the nuclear membrane dissolves and chromosomes move under microtubule control to align in metaphase. Paired chromosomes then separate to either pole of the cell in anaphase. Finally, two discrete nuclear membranes are formed in telophase.

21. **PLAP – seminoma.** CA 125 is a marker for ovarian cancer, CA 19-9 is a marker for pancreatic cancer, CA 15-3 is a tumour marker for breast cancer and CEA is a marker for a number of cancers, including bowel and cervical.

22. **The mode is a measure of data location.** Measures of location are the mode (most frequent), median (middle value) and mean (average). Measures of spread are range/interquartile range and standard deviation (spread of the mean). The median is the middle value of a data set and is used with ordinal data, while the mean is the average of a data set and may be used with ordinal but not nominal data.

23. **Optic nerve.** The internal carotid artery travels through the foramen lacerum, the facial nerve travels through the stylomastoid foramen and the vestibulocochlear and facial nerves through the internal acoustic meatus.

24. **Internal carotid artery.** The internal carotid artery passes through the carotid canal into the foramen lacerum.

25. **Abducens nerve.** The abducens nerve supplies the lateral rectus and runs through the medial wall of the cavernous sinus, in contact with the internal carotid artery. Cranial nerves III, IV, V_1 and V_2 run along the lateral wall of the cavernous sinus.

26. **Marginal mandibular branch of the facial nerve.** It supplies the circumoral musculature and runs below the angle of the mandible under platysma.

27. **The inferior lobe of the left lung is best auscultated posteriorly.** The pulmonary valve is auscultated in the left second intercostal space, the mitral in the fifth intercostal space, the midclavicular line on the left, and the tricuspid in the left parasternal fourth intercostal space. The left lung has two lobes, therefore only has an oblique fissure. The right horizontal fissure is in the fourth intercostal space. The right middle lobe is best heard anteriorly at the most inferior aspect of the chest wall.

28. **Sensation to the breast and nipple is from the 4th to the 6th intercostal nerve.** The thoracodorsal nerve supplies latissimus dorsi. Winging of the scapula is caused by weakness of the serratus anterior, which is supplied by the long thoracic nerve of Bell. The breast extends from the parasternal line to the midaxillary line, second to sixth rib. The axillary lymph nodes are divided into levels according to their relationship to the pectoralis minor and most of the breast drains to these.

29. **The jejunum is more vascular than the ileum.** Macroscopically, the difference between the jejunum and ileum is subtle. The jejunum is more vascular, hence pinker/darker red than the ileum. It has a larger lumen and longer vasa recta but shorter arcades (which can be viewed when holding the mesentery up to the light). Jejunal mesentery is also much less fatty.

30. **Serum calcium.** Hypercalcaemia can cause both pancreatitis and nephrocalcinosis.

31. **Three.** There are three compartments in the thigh: anterior (supplied by the femoral nerve), posterior (supplied by the sciatic nerve) and medial (supplied by the obturator nerve).

32. **Superior gluteal nerve.** The superior gluteal nerve supplies the

gluteus medius and minimis (hip abductors). When the leg is lifted on the contralateral side, the hip will drop on the side with the weak abductors, causing the Trendelenburg gait.

33. **There is a ~75% risk of further myocardial infarction intra-operatively.** Elective surgery should be cancelled then postponed for at least 6 months, if possible, to reduce the risk of re-infarction under anaesthesia.

34. **Amoxicillin/clavulanic acid.** The organism most commonly responsible for a UTI is *Escherichia coli*, therefore good Gram-negative cover is required when treating empirically. Trimethoprim is contained in trimethoprim/sulphamethoxazole and nitrofurantoin should be avoided in renal failure. Vancomycin and linezolid have good Gram-positive cover, so are not routinely used to treat UTIs unless indicated by the sensitivity of any organism cultured.

35. **Lactate >1.2 mmol/L.** 'Septic shock' is defined as refractory hypotension with a proven source of sepsis. Organ failure or dysfunction will follow unless corrected. Kidney dysfunction is seen in falling urine output. CNS dysfunction is seen in the GCS score and respiratory dysfunction is seen in hypoxia. 'Cardiovascular system dysfunction' is defined by rising lactate, suggesting tissue ischaemia.

36. **Central line.** This patient requires feeding, as she is malnourished (according to National Institute for Health and Clinical Excellence [NICE] guidelines). She has not eaten for more than 3 days but also has a bowel obstruction, therefore she requires TPN, as her gut will not be absorbing. If she ends up with <100 cm of small bowel, she will probably require lifelong TPN. (National Institute for Health and Clinical Excellence. Nutrition Support in Adults; oral nutrition support, enteral tube feeding and parenteral nutrition: NICE guideline 32. London: NIHCE; 2006. www.nice.org.uk/guidance/CG32)

37. **0.5 mL/kg/h**

38. **All of the above.** Hypernatraemia can be caused by water loss – for example, dehydration and diabetes insipidus – or excess salt retention, as in Conn's and Cushing's syndromes.

39. **Calcitonin.** Calcitonin is produced by parafollicular C cells in the

thyroid. It acts to reduce serum calcium by inhibiting bone resorption and stimulating renal excretion of calcium.

40. **Paget's disease of the nipple.** This is a malignant condition involving the nipple that looks like eczema. An underlying tumour is often, but not always, found, and an underlying breast lump may or may not be palpable.

41. **Increased pH.** Increased pH moves the curve to the left. Reduced pH, increased CO_2, increased temperature, increased 2,3-DPG and reduced tissue perfusion shift the curve to the right, promoting offloading of O_2 to the tissues.

42. **Respiratory alkalosis.** Initially, a respiratory alkalosis is seen due to hyperstimulation of the respiratory centre by aspirin. Eventually, an anion gap metabolic acidosis will occur.

43. **Lacunar ligament.** The borders of the femoral canal are: laterally, the lacunar ligament; medially, the femoral vein; anteriorly, the inguinal ligament; and, posteriorly, the pectineal ligament.

44. **Ovary.** CA 125 is a marker for ovarian cancer. It may also be raised in other malignant and benign conditions but is not 100% sensitive, thus is not useful as a screening test. However, a raised CA 125 may warrant further investigation, and the marker can be used for monitoring the response of an ovarian cancer to treatment.

45. **It is a risk factor for the development of bowel cancer.** Skip lesions are a feature of Crohn's disease, not of UC, which affects a continuous segment of bowel from the rectum proximal. Smoking is a positive risk factor for Crohn's but is protective against UC. UC affects the mucosa and submucosa only, whereas Crohn's affects the full thickness of the bowel. Crohn's disease is characterised by the presence of non-caseating granulomata. UC is a risk factor for the development of bowel cancer.

46. **Halfway between the pubic tubercle and the anterior superior iliac spine.** The deep ring is denoted by the midpoint of the inguinal ligament, which is halfway between the pubic tubercle and the anterior superior iliac spine. The mid-inguinal point, which lies halfway between the pubic symphysis and the anterior superior iliac spine,

indicates the location of the femoral pulse. The superficial ring lies above and medial to the pubic tubercle.

47. **Firstborn child.** Risk factors for developmental dysplasia of the hip include female sex, oligohydramnios, multiple pregnancy, breech position, firstborn child and prematurity. Certain ethnic groups are also more at risk, including Native Americans. There is a low incidence of the condition in babies of Chinese and African origin.

48. **T10.** Dermatomal distribution can vary, but the umbilical skin is most often in the T10 dermatome.

49. **50.0%.** FAP is inherited in an autosomal dominant pattern. This means that inheritance of a single affected allele is sufficient to cause the disease. If one parent is affected and the other is not, the risk of having an affected child is 50%.

50. **Anaplastic carcinoma.**

MRCS Part A Paper 1

Mock Paper 3

ANSWERS

1. **External carotid artery.** The external carotid is well away from the operation site and the common carotid is protected by the reflected strap muscles.

2. **Increased 2,3-DPG.** Factors causing a shift to the left include a decrease in temperature, decreased 2,3-DPG concentration, decreased CO_2 concentration and increased pH. Factors causing a shift to the right include an increase in temperature, increased 2,3-DPG concentration, increased CO_2 concentration and decreased pH. A shift to the left causes increased affinity of haemoglobin for O_2, making it easier to bind O_2 in the lung but more difficult to offload it at the tissues. A shift to the right causes decreased affinity of haemoglobin for O_2, making it easier to offload O_2 at the tissues. The 'Haldane effect' describes the relationship between the oxygenation of blood and its ability to carry CO_2.

3. **All of the above.** All answer options are primary lung cancers.

4. **Para-aortic.** The testes and ovaries drain to the para-aortic lymph nodes. This is because they start high up in the abdomen then migrate down during development, taking their lymph drainage and blood supply with them. In contrast, the scrotum drains to the inguinal lymph nodes.

5. **Gastroduodenal artery.** As the gastroduodenal artery lies posterior

to the first part of the duodenum, it is at risk of erosion by peptic ulcers located on the posterior duodenal wall.

6. **The size of the primary tumour, the grade of the tumour and the involvement of lymph nodes.** These are the three components of the Nottingham Prognostic Index, which is used to estimate the prognosis of a malignant breast tumour. It is used to help determine which patients would benefit from adjuvant treatment.

7. **Saphenous nerve.** The saphenous nerve supplies sensation to the medial aspect of the foot and lower leg. In runs in close proximity to the long saphenous vein, thus can be damaged in stripping. Patients should be informed of this risk at the time of consent.

8. **Palmar cutaneous branch of the median nerve.** The palmar cutaneous branch of the median nerve supplies sensation to the thenar eminence. The recurrent branch of the median nerve is the motor supply to the thenar muscles – the opponens pollicis, abductor pollicis brevis and flexor pollicis brevis (the lumbricals are supplied by an earlier branch of the median nerve).

9. **4.0–4.5 kPa.** CO_2 is a potent cerebral vasodilator, so $PaCO_2$ should be kept between 4.0 and 4.5 kPa to reduce the risk of raised intracranial pressure (ICP) and secondary brain injury from cerebral ischaemia.

10. **Chest infection.** This patient has features of a systemic inflammatory response in keeping with possible sepsis. He has desaturated and, as a smoker, he is at increased risk of chest sepsis, particularly following a period of relative immobilisation associated with an orthopaedic operation.

11. **Insulin-like growth factor.** Insulin-like-growth factors are from a family of proteins stimulated by growth hormone. They are involved in organ development and regeneration. All the other answer options are involved in wound healing and granulation tissue formation.

12. *Treponema pallidum.* This is the organism that causes syphilis. It can present at different stages and tertiary syphilis occurs in about one third of patients who are not treated. It is rare in the United Kingdom but may cause aortitis due to inflammation of the arterial tunica media.

13. **Choroid plexus tumour.** A choroid plexus tumour may cause either

a communicating hydrocephalus (via the overproduction of cerebrospinal fluid) or non-communicating hydrocephalus (via physical obstruction of the ventricular system). All of the other answer options cause a non-communicating obstructive hydrocephalus.

14. **Joint subluxation.** Joint subluxation is characteristic of rheumatoid arthritis on X-ray. Subchondral cysts, subchondral sclerosis and osteophytes are typically seen in osteoarthritis. Pathological fractures are associated with osteoporosis and malignancy, among other pathologies.

15. **Pulmonary stenosis.** Tetralogy of Fallot is characterised by four abnormalities: ventricular septal defect, overriding aorta, pulmonary stenosis and right ventricular hypertrophy. It is the most common cause of cyanotic congenital cardiac disease.

16. **Conn's syndrome.** Conn's syndrome (primary hyperaldosteronism) causes hypertension via renal salt and water reabsorption. Addison's disease (chronic adrenal insufficiency) may cause hypotension. Sheehan's syndrome is hypopituitarism associated with hypovolaemia during childbirth. Waterhouse–Friderichsen syndrome is acute hypoadrenalism due to adrenal haemorrhage (usually secondary to infection). Diabetes insipidus causes an inability to concentrate urine, which may lead to dehydration and hypotension.

17. **Hashimoto's thyroiditis.** Hashimoto's thyroiditis is characterised by the presence of serum thyroid peroxidase antibodies. Graves' disease is characterised by the presence of TSH receptor-stimulating antibodies. De Quervain's thyroiditis is rare and secondary to viral infection. Subacute lymphocytic thyroiditis is autoimmune and often asymptomatic.

18. **SIADH.** SIADH causes hyponatraemia with euvolaemia, as total body water is increased but sodium level stays the same (i.e. it is a dilutional hyponatraemia). As such, serum osmolality is reduced while urine osmolality is raised (as urine is hyperconcentrated).

19. **It is the most common intra-abdominal tumour of childhood.** Wilms' tumour is the most common intra-abdominal tumour of childhood and is more common in children than adults. Only 5% are bilateral. Five-year survival is approximately 90%. It is

treated primarily by surgical excision and/or chemotherapy and/or radiotherapy.

20. **Caeruloplasmin.** Caeruloplasmin binds copper in plasma. Albumin binds calcium, among other things; haptoglobin binds free haemoglobin; apolipoprotein binds lipids; and transferrin binds iron.

21. **Plasma cells produce antibodies against the persistent antigen.** Macrophages are the predominant cell type in chronic inflammation. IL-1 activates fibroblasts. IL-6 and TNF-alpha are pyrogens, which are part of the acute inflammatory response. TGF-beta stimulates fibrosis. T helper cells activate B lymphocytes to produce plasma cells.

22. **Medullary carcinoma is derived from C cells.** On FNA (which is cytological and does not involve histology), follicular carcinoma is virtually indistinguishable from follicular adenoma. Sixty per cent of thyroid carcinomas are papillary, making these the most common thyroid malignancy. Aside from anaplastic carcinoma, thyroid carcinomas rarely metastasise. Medullary thyroid cancer is associated with MEN 2.

23. *Tityus trinitatis.* *Tityus trinitatis* is a scorpion found in Trinidad whose sting may cause acute pancreatitis.

24. **Microtubules.** Microtubules forming on the mitotic spindle control the movement of chromosomes to the pole of the cell during mitosis.

25. **If a study is adequately powered, this lessens the chance of obtaining a false-negative result.** Non-parametric tests are used for non-normally distributed data, while parametric tests are used to assess normally distributed data. 'Sensitivity' refers to the ability of a test to correctly identify those with a disease, while 'specificity' is the ability of a test to correctly identify those who do not have a disease. A 'type I error' occurs when a test identifies a difference between two sets of data that does not exist (i.e. a false positive), while a 'type II error' occurs when a test identifies no difference between two sets of data when in fact there is a difference (i.e. a false negative). 'Correlation' is a measure of the strength of association between two variables, while 'confounding' occurs when another variable influences a test's results.

26. **Spinal roots of the accessory nerve.** The glossopharyngeal nerve,

spinal roots of the accessory nerve and the medulla oblongata pass through the foramen magnum. The facial nerve passes through the stylomastoid foramen. The trigeminal nerve passes through the foramen ovale.

27. **Trochlear.** A fourth cranial nerve palsy is difficult to diagnose. Patients cannot turn their eye downward when it is rotated medially, thus descending stairs is difficult. Tilting the head allows compensation for this palsy and relieves the double vision.

28. **Great auricular.** It originates from C2–3 and supplies sensation to the skin over the parotid, mastoid, outer ear and angle of the jaw.

29. **Expiration is essentially a passive process involving relaxation of the diaphragm and elastic recoil of the lungs.** The diaphragm is supplied by the phrenic nerve (C3, 4 and 5) and is the most important muscle of respiration. Contraction of the diaphragm increases intra-thoracic volume, which reduces the intra-thoracic pressure below atmospheric pressure so that air is sucked in. The intercostal muscles are supplied by their respective spinal roots and are used more in forced respiration. Pump-handle movement describes the changes in antero-posterior diameter that occur predominantly in the upper half of the ribcage during ventilation. Bucket-handle movement describes the changes in transverse diameter that occur predominantly in the lower half of the ribcage during ventilation. These lower ribs have no sternal attachment so can't be described as vertebro-sternal. Expiration is passive, involving relaxation of the diaphragm and elastic recoil of the lungs.

30. **The subclavian vein runs between the subclavius and anterior scalene muscles.** The subclavian vein runs in front of the subclavian artery, covered by the scalenus anterior. Subclavius and the clavicular head of the pectoralis major muscle are anterior to the vein. The thoracic duct drains into the left venous angle. The external jugular vein drains directly into the subclavian vein.

31. **Thoracodorsal.** Weakness of the latissimus dorsi (responsible for adduction and internal rotation of the arm) is from damage to the thoracodorsal nerve (a branch of the posterior cord of the brachial plexus) running on the posterior wall of the axilla.

32. **The median nerve is situated medial to the brachial artery.** The contents of the cubital fossa are (lateral to medial): biceps tendon, brachial artery and median nerve. The boundaries are: floor, brachialis; roof, deep fascia of the forearm; medially, pronator teres; and, laterally, brachioradialis.

33. **Uterine artery.** The ureter inserts into the bladder in an oblique fashion at the postero-lateral surface of the bladder. Before it enters the bladder, it is anteriorly crossed by the uterine artery in females and the vas deferens in males.

34. **Extradural haematoma.** The middle meningeal artery runs outside of the dura (to supply it). Subdural haematomas are usually venous bleeds and subarachnoid haemorrhages occur within the subarachnoid space (e.g. berry aneurysm of the Circle of Willis).

35. **Pneumatic compression devices on the legs.** Gel cushions are used to reduce pressure-sore formation. Wrapping the arms protects them in the paralysed patient and keeps them out of the surgical field. The Bair Hugger® is for patient warming. Mechanical VTE prophylaxis is used in theatre and pharmacological prophylaxis is usually delayed until at least 6 hours post-operative.

36. **Amikacin.** Erythromycin is a macrolide and has a similar antibacterial spectrum to penicillin. Vancomycin and teicoplanin are glycopeptides that work against aerobic and anaerobic Gram-positive organisms. Linezolid is an oxazolidinone with Gram-positive cover used for methicillin-resistant *Staphylococcus aureus* and vancomycin-resistant enterococci.

37. **Vitamin E.** Vitamins A, D, E and K are fat soluble.

38. **Physiological stress response.** In the first 24–36 hours, the body's response to stress is to release glucocorticoids and mineralocorticoids, which stimulate sodium and water retention. It should also be noted that anaesthetics cause ADH release and further water retention.

39. **All of the above.** These all affect a patient's ability to ventilate their lung fully through deep breathing.

40. **Mammography and FNA.** Although clinically you presume this lump to be fat necrosis, and the history is consistent with this, all patients presenting with a breast lump should undergo triple assessment, as you

do not want to miss identifying a breast carcinoma. As this woman is over the age of 35, mammography is the imaging technique of choice.

41. **Affects both preload and afterload.** The creation of a pneumoperitoneum causes an increase in intra-abdominal pressure. This compresses the great veins, causing an initial increase followed by a decrease in preload. Compression of arteries causes an increase in peripheral vascular resistance and afterload.

42. **Non-selective COX inhibition.** Ibuprofen is a non-selective COX inhibitor, inhibiting the actions of both COX-1 and COX-2. COX is an enzyme that converts arachidonic acid to prostaglandins. It is thought that COX-2 inhibition is responsible for the anti-inflammatory effects of ibuprofen, whereas COX-1 inhibition is responsible for many of the side effects.

43. **2 cm below and lateral to the pubic tubercle.**

44. **Trochlear nerve.** The trochlear nerve supplies the superior oblique muscle, which is responsible for moving the eye downwards when it is rotated medially. This movement is important when looking down stairs or reading a book. The abducens nerve supplies the lateral rectus muscle, which is responsible for lateral movement of the eye. The oculomotor nerve supplies the remaining muscles of the eye. The optic nerve transmits visual information from the eye, and the facial nerve supplies the muscles involved in making facial expressions.

45. **Protamine.** Protamine binds heparin to form a complex that has no anticoagulant action.

46. **Median nerve.** The median nerve passes anterior to the elbow joint, medial to the brachial artery in the cubital fossa. Like the brachial artery, it can be easily damaged at this point by a supracondylar fracture of the humerus. Sensation to the hand is supplied by a combination of the median, ulnar and radial nerves, but the thenar eminence is supplied by the median nerve.

47. **External laryngeal.** The cricothyroid muscle acts to tighten the vocal cords, enabling high-pitched singing. It is the only muscle of the larynx that is not supplied by the recurrent laryngeal nerve. The external laryngeal nerve is a branch of the superior laryngeal nerve, which is a branch of the vagus nerve.

48. **Common hepatic.** The free edge of the lesser omentum contains the portal triad. This consists of the portal vein, the common hepatic artery and the common bile duct. Compression of the vessels at this point to control bleeding is known as 'Pringle's manoeuvre'.

49. *Staphylococcus aureus.* *Staphylococcus aureus* is the most common organism found in osteomyelitis.

50. **Common peroneal.** The sciatic nerve is formed from the nerve roots L4 to S1 and divides into the tibial nerve and the common peroneal nerve, usually in the popliteal fossa. The common peroneal nerve winds around the neck of the fibula and is vulnerable to injury there. It divides into deep and superficial branches. The deep peroneal nerve supplies the muscles required for dorsiflexion and provides sensation to the third web space. The superficial peroneal nerve supplies the muscles required for eversion and sensation to the lateral leg and dorsum of the foot. Inversion is provided by the tibialis posterior and the tibial nerve (and also by tibialis anterior which is supplied by the deep peroneal nerve). The correct answer is the common peroneal nerve as function of both superficial and deep peroneal nerves is lost, but that of the tibial nerve remains intact.

MRCS Part A Paper 1

Mock Paper 4

ANSWERS

1. **Clonidine.** Clonidine is a centrally acting alpha-2 agonist. Frusemide is a loop diuretic, spironolactone is a potassium-sparing diuretic and amlodipine and diltiazem are calcium channel blockers.

2. **All of the above.** All of the named hormones are produced by the adrenal cortex.

3. **Anaplastic carcinoma.** Anaplastic carcinoma has a 5-year survival rate of <10%. Papillary, follicular and medullary thyroid cancer have a 5-year survival rate of 96%, 91% and 83%, respectively. Follicular adenomata are benign. (Cancer Research UK. Thyroid cancer survival statistics. www.cancerresearchuk.org/cancer-info/cancerstats/types/thyroid/survival/thyroid-cancer-survival-statistics)

4. *Streptococcus viridans.* Bacterial endocarditis is most commonly caused by Group A streptococci, *Pseudomonas* and the HACEK group (*Haemophilus parainfluenzae*, *Aggregatibacter*, *Cardiobacterium hominis*, *Eikenella corrodens* and *Kingella kingae*).

5. **The posterior border is formed by the peritoneum over the inferior vena cava.** The epiploic foramen is the entry portal to the lesser sac. Anteriorly, it is bordered by the free edge of the lesser omentum, containing the portal triad. Posterior is the inferior vena cava with its overlying peritoneum. Superior is the caudate process of the liver (with overlying peritoneum) and inferior is the stomach and the first part of the duodenum (with overlying peritoneum).

6. **Renal vein, renal artery, ureter.**

7. **Parietal cells in the stomach.** Intrinsic factor is secreted by parietal cells, which are found in the stomach. Intrinsic factor is required for vitamin B12 absorption in the small bowel. G cells in the stomach produce gastrin. Enterochromaffin-like cells are found in the stomach and produce histamine.

8. **Breastfeeding a child for more than 6 months.** Lactation is a protective rather than risk factor. Women who have more oestrogen exposure are at an increased risk of developing breast cancer. Therefore, risk factors include early menarche, late menopause, taking the combined oral contraceptive pill and receiving hormone replacement therapy. Nulliparity is also a risk factor. Having a first pregnancy at a young age is protective, but women who have their first pregnancy aged 35 or over have a greater risk than those who remain nulliparous. Further risk factors include a personal or family history of breast cancer.

9. **Radial.** The radial nerve runs in the radial groove, spiralling around the posterior aspect of the shaft of the humerus. As such, it can be damaged in mid-shaft humeral fractures. Power grip requires extension of the wrist and the radial nerve supplies all the muscles of wrist extension. The ulnar nerve is intact and this supplies the small muscles of the hand responsible for finger adduction and abduction.

10. **Lateral cutaneous nerve of the thigh.** The lateral cutaneous nerve of the thigh arises from the lateral border of the psoas (L2–3 divisions) and runs inferiorly toward the anterior superior iliac spine, where it runs beneath the inguinal ligament into the thigh to supply sensation to its lateral aspect. It can be damaged during inguinal hernia repairs and any such damage may result in patients reporting pain and numbness of the lateral aspect of the thigh. The condition is known as 'meralgia paraesthetica'.

11. **Supraspinatus.** The supraspinatus is responsible for the initiation of abduction from 0 to 15 degrees. After this, the action of the deltoid enables abduction. When the supraspinatus is torn or diseased, patients have difficulty initiating abduction. They may compensate by either leaning their torso over to that side or using the other arm to help initiate the movement.

12. **30 degrees head up.** Thirty degrees head up is considered the optimum position for nursing patients with head injuries in order to prevent raised ICP and secondary brain injury from cerebral ischaemia.

13. **Catheterise and measure hourly urine output.** This patient is unwell with features of SIRS. His fluid balance should be carefully monitored and this necessitates the insertion of a catheter and hourly urine output measurements.

14. **3–5 years.**

15. **Antithrombin III deficiency.** Antithrombin III deficiency is an autosomal dominant hypercoaguability disorder. Protein S and protein C deficiencies also cause hypercoaguability. Antiphospholipid antibody production is a secondary cause of hypercoaguability.

16. **Autosomal recessive polycystic kidney disease.** Ehlers–Danlos syndrome, Marfan's syndrome, NF1, coarctation of the aorta and autosomal dominant polycystic kidney disease are all associated with an increased occurrence of berry aneurysm formation. However, autosomal recessive polycystic kidney disease is not.

17. **Reduced FEV_1.** Obstructive lung diseases, such as COPD, are characterised by a low/normal vital capacity, reduced FEV_1, reduced FEV_1/FVC ratio and reduced PEFR. Restrictive lung diseases, such as pulmonary fibrosis, are characterised by reduced vital capacity, reduced FEV_1, normal or increased FEV_1/FVC ratio and normal PEFR.

18. **Small-cell carcinoma is usually treated with chemotherapy.** Adenocarcinoma usually arises peripherally. With surgical resection (in non-small-cell lung cancer), survival is >50% at 5 years. Without surgical resection, prognosis is poor. Small-cell lung cancer is most commonly associated with paraneoplastic syndromes. All forms of lung cancer may not be symptomatic and may present incidentally.

19. **Prostate cancer metastases to bone are sclerotic.** Adenocarcinoma is the most common form of prostate cancer and usually found in the peripheral zone of the prostate. The PSA level increases with age and there is no specific cut-off point to diagnose cancer, as there are a number of reasons why PSA may be raised. Lung cancer is the leading

cause of death from cancer in men, as many men with prostate cancer do not die from the disease.

20. **Hypocalcaemia occurs because of lipid saponification.** The reference range for serum amylase is 40–140 U/L and a raised amylase level in the absence of symptoms of acute pancreatitis is not necessarily diagnostic of acute pancreatitis. The evidence for antibiotics in acute pancreatitis is equivocal. Necrosis is a delayed complication of acute pancreatitis. Patients may require insulin therapy, but this will be due to beta cell damage.

21. **Bcl-2.** Bcl-2 is an example of a gene regulating programmed cell death. p53 and APC are examples of tumour suppressor genes – they are responsible for halting cell division but, when mutated, are down regulated and no longer act as tumour suppressors. Ras and ERB-1 are examples of oncogenes. When mutated, they promote cell division.

22. **Pregnancy.** Pregnancy causes venous stasis due to pelvic vein obstruction. It also causes hypercoaguability. Factor V Leiden, protein C deficiency and malignancy all cause hypercoaguability.

23. ***Pneumocystis carinii* is described as both a fungus and a protozoa.** Aflatoxin is produced by *Aspergillus* fungi. Oesophageal *Candida* infection is typically painful. *Histoplasma* species are visible to the human eye as they grow as mycelia that look brown. *Aspergillus* species usually cause an aspergilloma that looks similar on X-ray to a tuberculoma in that they are both cavitating lung lesions, but the immunological response of each differs.

24. **Platelets.** Platelets release prostaglandins, leukotrienes, histamine and serotonin and synthesise thromboxane A_2.

25. **Lymphocytes predominate in autoimmune disease.** Lymphocytes are the predominant cell type in viral and autoimmune infections; neutrophils in bacterial infections; eosinophils in allergic reactions and parasites; plasma cells in spirochaetal infections (e.g. Lyme disease and syphilis); and macrophages in typhoid, TB and fungal infections.

26. **Facial nerve.** The glossopharyngeal nerve travels through the jugular foramen, the abducens nerve through the superior orbital fissure,

the optic nerve through the sphenoid bone and the mandibular branch of the trigeminal through the sphenoid bone.

27. **Chorda tympani.** The facial nerve branches in the facial canal. The greater petrosal nerve supplies the lacrimal gland, the nerve to the stapedius supplies the stapedius muscle and the chorda tympani is responsible for taste to the anterior two-thirds of the tongue, as well as parasympathetic innervation to the salivary and submandibular glands. It also provides some sensory supply to the tympanic membrane. The auricular nerve supplies sensation to the skin around the external auditory meatus. The lingual nerve is a branch of the mandibular division of the trigeminal nerve (sensory).

28. **Oculomotor.** This cluster of symptoms is a third cranial nerve palsy. It has multiple aetiologies, including head trauma.

29. **The endothoracic fascia is adherent to the inner thoracic cage between the innermost intercostal muscle and parietal pleura.** A chest drain is usually inserted in the 4th–6th intercostal space, anterior to the midaxillary line. Needle decompression of a tension pneumothorax is performed in the second intercostal space at the midclavicular line. The neurovascular bundle runs along the inferior edge of the aspect of the rib in the plane between the internal and innermost intercostals.

30. **It contains lymphocytes and Hassall's corpuscles.** The thymus is a gland separate to the thyroid that contains lymphocytes and thymocytes (Hassall's corpuscles). It usually atrophies before puberty and sits in front of the heart. It is responsible for T cell development.

31. **Plantaris.** The Achilles tendon is the common calcaneal insertion of the gastrocnemius, soleus and plantaris.

32. **Middle meningeal artery.** It supplies the dura mater.

33. **Over an area with a good blood supply.** It is the surgeon's ultimate responsibility to check where the monopolar diathermy plate is sited, although it is something often done by theatre staff. The plate should be placed away from metal work and bony prominences, on an area with a good blood supply that is hair-free for good plate contact. Alcohol is flammable, so the use of an alcohol skin preparation should be avoided near the diathermy plate due to the risk of fire.

34. **It is a vitamin K antagonist.** Vitamin K deficiency affects clotting factors II, VII, IX and X, thus Vitamin K is warfarin's reversal agent. Warfarin requires continuous monitoring and re-dosing. Direct factor Xa agents include rivaroxaban. LMWH and unfractionated heparin bind to antithrombin III. Direct thrombin inhibitors include dabigatran.

35. **Prolene™.** To prevent turbulent flow and minimise intimal injury within the artery, a monofilament suture is used. Further, as it is an artery, a non-absorbable monofilament is selected.

36. **1 mmol/kg/L.**

37. **All of the above.**

38. **As hydroxyapatite.** Almost all calcium is found in bone as hydroxyapatite. A small amount is found as calcium phosphate salt.

39. **All of the above.** CO_2, protons and 2,3-DPG all reduce haemoglobin's affinity for O_2, therefore shifting the O_2–haemoglobin dissociation curve to the right (the Bohr effect), enabling O_2 to be offloaded to the tissues.

40. **0–10 mmHg.** 'CVP' is the pressure in the right atrium. It is not a useful figure on its own. The trend of CVP in response to a fluid challenge can determine circulating volume (when there is no cardiac or pulmonary dysfunction altering the reading).

41. **Recurrent laryngeal.** The recurrent laryngeal nerve runs very close to branches of the inferior thyroid artery and can be damaged during surgery involving this vessel. The recurrent laryngeal nerve supplies all of the intrinsic muscles of the larynx apart from the cricothyroid.

42. **Crohn's disease.** Non-caseating granulomata are characteristic of Crohn's disease.

43. **Inferior edge of the liver, common hepatic duct, cystic duct.** The superior border is the inferior edge of the liver, the medial border is the common hepatic duct and the lateral border is the cystic duct.

44. **Small bowel can be identified on plain radiograph by the presence of valvulae conniventes.** The first part of the duodenum is retroperitoneal. The rest of the small bowel is intra-peritoneal. Distal to the second part of the duodenum, the small bowel is supplied by the superior mesenteric artery. Proximal to this, the blood supply

comes from the coeliac axis. The small bowel mesentery runs from the DJ flexure to the right iliac fossa. The large bowel can be identified at operation by the presence of taeniae coli whereas the small bowel does not have these. The small bowel can be identified on plain X-ray by the presence of valvulae conniventes, which appear as opaque lines travelling all the way across the bowel lumen.

45. **Lung carcinoma.** Lung carcinoma is the most common fatal cancer in both women and men in the United Kingdom. Breast carcinoma is the most common cancer to affect women but is responsible for fewer cancer deaths than lung cancer.

46. **Follicular thyroid carcinoma.** Follicular thyroid carcinoma is not part of MEN 1.

47. **24 hours.** The healthy neonate delivered at term should pass meconium within 24 hours.

48. **Haemoglobin concentration.** The O_2–haemoglobin dissociation curve reflects the affinity of a single haemoglobin molecule for O_2, so is unaffected by haemoglobin concentration.

49. **11.** She scores 4 for having her eyes open, 3 for inappropriate speech and 4 for flexing in response to pain.

50. **Insertion of a surgical chest drain in the left hemithorax.** As this patient's clinical signs are consistent with a massive haemothorax on the left, insertion of a surgical chest drain on the left is warranted. She is not stable enough for a chest X-ray and has no clinical suggestion of cardiac tamponade. As she is talking, her airway is currently patent and this means that endotracheal intubation is not indicated as your *first* management step.

MRCS Part A Paper 1

Mock Paper 5

ANSWERS

1. **Labetalol.** All are beta-blockers. As labetalol also has alpha-blocking effects, it is used to treat hypertension in phaeochromocytoma, which results from increased circulating catecholamines.

2. **All of the above.** Infective endocarditis typically causes regurgitant valve disease.

3. **Gastrinoma.** Ductal adenocarcinoma is the most common form of pancreatic cancer but is not neuroendocrine in origin. Insulinomas and glucagonomas are neuroendocrine tumours of the islet cells. A gastrinoma may derive from the duodenum or the pancreas. A somatostatinoma is a tumour of the delta cells of the endocrine pancreas.

4. **Neck of the pancreas.** The trans-pyloric plane is a transverse plane at the level of L1. This is a point halfway between the sternal notch and the pubic symphysis. Structures situated on the trans-pyloric plane include the fundus of the gallbladder, the neck of the pancreas, the DJ flexure, the end of the spinal cord, the hilum of the left kidney, the upper pole of the right kidney, the origin of the superior mesenteric artery, the pylorus of the stomach and the first part of the duodenum.

5. **Gastrin release from a neuroendocrine tumour.** In Zollinger–Ellison syndrome, a gastrinoma in the pancreas or small bowel produces excess gastrin. This causes increased production of stomach acid, leading to peptic ulceration.

6. **Adenocarcinoma is most commonly situated in the lower third of the oesophagus.** The incidence of adenocarcinoma of the oesophagus is increasing in the United Kingdom and it is now more common than squamous-cell carcinoma of the oesophagus. It usually occurs in the lower third of the oesophagus, near the gastro-oesophageal junction. Its main risk factor is Barrett's oesophagus, which can become dysplastic. The main risk factors for squamous-cell carcinoma of the oesophagus are smoking and drinking alcohol.

7. **Dorsum of foot, just lateral to the extensor hallucis longus and posterior border of the medial malleolus.** The two foot pulses that are commonly palpated are the dorsalis pedis and the posterior tibial artery. The dorsalis pedis can be found lateral to the extensor hallucis longus tendon (you can ask the patient to lift up their big toe to demonstrate this). The posterior tibial artery can be found behind the medial malleolus. This is also where you should direct your Doppler probe if you are not able to palpate the pulses.

8. **Supraspinatus.** Supraspinatus pathology is often characterised by a 'painful arc', in which the patient complains of pain when abducting the arm between 60 and 120 degrees. The most common is supraspinatus tendonitis, in which the inflamed tendon is pressed against the acromium during this part of abduction. It can also occur when the tendon has a partial tear.

9. **70 mmHg.** Cerebral perfusion pressure (CPP) = MAP − ICP. Ideally, MAP is kept around 70 mmHg to maintain CPP and prevent secondary brain injury from cerebral ischaemia.

10. **1.5–2.5 L water and 50–100 mmol/L sodium; 40–80 mmol/L potassium.** The March 2011 GIFTASUP guidelines state that, to meet maintenance requirements, patients should receive 50–100 mmol/L of sodium and 40–80 mmol/L potassium in 1.5–2.5 L of fluid daily. (Anaesthesia UK. British consensus guidelines on intravenous fluid therapy for adult surgical patients. GIFTASUP; 2009. www.renal.org/pages/media/download_gallery/GIFTASUP%20 FINAL_05_01_09.pdf)

11. **Deep vein thrombosis.** This patient has multiple risk factors for

deep vein thrombosis, including her immobilisation during a long-haul flight, her receipt of hormone replacement therapy and the fact that she smokes. The insect bite is unlikely to be the cause, as there are no other features of infection. Unilateral leg swelling with a background of risk factors for VTE must be investigated as such.

12. **Woven bone.** There are three main stages in fracture healing:

    1. the reactive phase, in which haematoma forms and there is an influx of cells in response to the inflammation

    2. the reparative phase, in which haematoma is organised into granulation tissue, callus is formed and woven bone is laid down, then mineralisation begins the conversion of woven bone into lamellar bone

    3. the remodelling phase, during which osteoclastic activity forms compact bone.

13. *Escherichia coli.* Meningitis-causing bacteria in neonates include *Escherichia coli*, Group B streptococcus and *Listeria monocytogenes*. *Neisseria meningitides* and *Haemophilus influenzae* are common pathogens in infants and young adults.

14. *Staphylococcus aureus.* *Staphylococcus aureus* is the most common organism responsible for breast abscesses in both lactating and non-lactating women.

15. **Nuclear pleomorphism.** Malignant cells are typically poorly differentiated, with a high nuclear/cytoplasmic ratio (due to the increased rate of cell division). They also have a high number of mitoses and hyperchromatism.

16. **Smoking.** 'Virchow's triad' refers to the three components of thrombosis: hypercoaguability, venous stasis/turbulence and endothelial injury. Smoking causes hypercoaguability.

17. **Standard deviation is a measure of data spread.** Sex and ethnicity are examples of nominal data; age and GCS score are examples of ordinal data. The median is the middle value of a data set. Weight and height are continuous variables.

18. **Acute glomerulonephritis is an example of a type III reaction.** Myasthenia is an example of a type V reaction while anaphylaxis is a

type I reaction. Type IV reactions are cell mediated and type II reactions are antibody mediated.

19. **Preoperative shaving can increase the incidence of wound infection.** Wound infections are still usually bacterial; however, immunocompromised patients are at high risk of fungal infection, so are often started on dual (empirical) therapy with an antibiotic and antifungal agent.

20. **There is evidence of healing with angiogenesis.** 'Chronic inflammation' is infiltration of monocytes, lymphocytes and plasma cells causing ongoing tissue destruction. Its classification requires evidence of healing through fibroblastic activity, angiogenesis and scar formation (which initially involves type III collagen that is then replaced with type I as the scar matures). Causative agents include autoimmune and granulomatous diseases (e.g. TB).

21. **The petrous temporal bone transmits the lesser petrosal nerve.** The vestibulocochlear nerve and facial nerve travel in the internal acoustic meatus, part of the petrous temporal bone, which also transmits the lesser and greater petrosal nerves, which emerge through its antero-superior surface. The abducens nerve runs through the superior orbital fissure and the zygomatic nerve runs through the zygoma.

22. **Mandibular.** The facial nerve divides into five branches within the parotid gland: the temporal branch, which raises the eyebrows; the zygomatic branch, which closes the eyes tightly; the buccal branch, which blows out the cheeks; the mandibular branch, which bears the teeth; and the cervical branch, which tenses the platysma. Therefore, the facial nerve supplies the muscles of facial expression.

23. **Downward and medial.** The inferior rectus muscle is often entrapped in the 'blowout' (orbital floor) fracture. This restricts the downward and medial movements of the eye.

24. **The lung under the anterior surface of the left chest wall is predominantly upper lobe.** The trachea bifurcates at the manubriosternal angle (angle of Louis – T4/5). The right main bronchus is larger in diameter and forms less of an angle with the trachea, meaning that foreign objects are most likely to lodge there. The right lung has three lobes, whereas the left lung has two.

25. **The thoracic aorta runs in both the inferior and superior mediastina.** The ascending aorta gives off coronary artery branches at its origin. The descending thoracic aorta is related posteriorly to the left main bronchus and issues posterior intercostal arterial branches. It crosses the diaphragm at T12.

26. **The medial breast is supplied by branches from the anterior intercostal arteries.** The breast has four sources of arterial blood. The internal thoracic artery provides the anterior intercostal arteries, which supply the medial breast. The lateral breast is supplied by the lateral thoracic artery. The superior epigastric artery branches from the internal thoracic artery and supplies the rectus muscle. Deep perforators come from the thoracoacromial trunk (a branch of the axillary artery).

27. **Second part of the duodenum.** The second, third and fourth parts of the duodenum are retroperitoneal. The tail of the pancreas is intraperitoneal, as it sits in the splenic hilum.

28. **Four.** There are four compartments in the leg: the anterior, containing the deep peroneal nerve and anterior tibial vessels; the lateral, containing the superficial peroneal nerve; the deep posterior, containing the tibial nerve and posterior tibial vessels; and the superficial posterior, containing the sural nerve.

29. **Four.** The pterion is the junction of the frontal, parietal, temporal and sphenoid bones.

30. **The most common cause of accidental burns is misapplication of the diathermy plate.** It is a common misconception that most burns occur when the surgeon slips. In bipolar instruments, the active and return electrodes are within the instrument (e.g. forceps). However, in monopolar diathermy, the active electrode is within the instrument and the return electrode is the plate. As with all electrical appliances, diathermy uses alternating current, so use of an alcohol preparation increases the risk of surgical fires. The presence of an implantable cardioverter-defibrillator and/or pacemaker is a relative contraindication to diathermy.

31. **All of the above.** The lungs regulate $PaCO_2$ levels. The blood contains plasma proteins and haemoglobin for buffering. The kidney

regulates proton and bicarbonate excretion. The liver generates bicarbonate and ammonium in glutamine metabolism.

32. **Flumazenil.** Naloxone reverses morphine. Protamine reverses heparin. Intralipid® reverses local anaesthetic.

33. **Trans-thoracic echocardiogram.** Other examples of non-invasive cardiac assessment include ECG, sphygmomanometry and pulse oximetry.

34. **Protamine is the reversal agent.** LMWH binds and accelerates antithrombin III activity, which prevents factors X and II from catalysing thrombin formation (required for clot formation). It is usually administered subcutaneously and does not require monitoring. Warfarin acts on vitamin K-dependent factors II, VII, IX and X and is an oral agent that requires monitoring. Similarly, heparin binds antithrombin III. Direct thrombin inhibitors (e.g. dabigatran) and factor Xa inhibitors (e.g. rivaroxaban) are also oral agents that do not require monitoring.

35. **Refractory pulmonary oedema.** Fluid overload that does not respond to diuretic therapy and fluid restriction will require haemofiltration (which is better at removing fluid than haemodialysis). Other indications for dialysis include hyperkalaemia, uraemia (Ur >30 mmol/L), creatinine clearance <10 mmol/L and signs of encephalopathy.

36. **All of the above.** TUR of the prostate syndrome causes iatrogenic water excess. SIADH causes water retention, whereas nephrotic syndrome causes sodium and water retention, with the net outcome being hyponatraemia. Diarrhoea can cause hyponatraemia through excessive salt and water loss but with even greater sodium loss.

37. **Capnography.** Ventilation is a measure of how well CO_2 is expelled. Therefore, capnography is the only accurate measurement. Pulse oximetry measures arterial O_2 saturations.

38. **Proton pump inhibitor.** This patient is critically ill, thus susceptible to stress ulcers occurring in gastric and duodenal mucosa due to the body's physiological response to stress. A proton pump inhibitor should be considered in all critically ill surgical patients to protect against upper GI bleeds.

39. **Appendices epiploicae are features of the large bowel rather than the small bowel.** The caecum is the most distensible part of the large bowel. On plain radiograph, the small bowel can be identified by the presence of lines crossing the whole diameter of the bowel, whereas the large bowel can be identified by lines crossing only part of the diameter of the bowel. The rectum is rarely affected by ischaemia due to its good blood supply. Adenocarcinoma is the most common form of large bowel malignancy.

40. **Increased vitamin D activation in the kidney.** PTH is released in response to low serum calcium levels. It influences calcium levels by acting on bone, intestine and the kidneys. Increased PTH results in activation of osteoclastic activity, enabling the release of calcium and phosphate from bone. In the kidney, PTH causes increased phosphate excretion and calcium reabsorption. The kidney is also responsible for one stage of vitamin D activation, and this is increased. In the intestine, PTH causes increased absorption of both calcium and phosphate.

41. **Stomach.** The stomach and lesser omentum lie anterior to the lesser sac.

42. **Hodgkin's lymphoma.** Reed–Sternberg cells are large bi- or multi-nucleated cells that are found in Hodgkin's lymphoma.

43. **Reduced appetite.** The other answer options are features of hyperthyroidism.

44. **Ramipril.** Ramipril is an angiotensin-converting enzyme inhibitor. Angiotensin-converting enzyme is responsible for the conversion of angiotensin I to angiotensin II. Inhibition of this enzyme leads to a reduction in angiotensin II, which in turn leads to a reduction in aldosterone. Aldosterone causes increased potassium excretion, so a reduction in aldosterone can lead to hyperkalaemia. Potassium-sparing diuretics such as spironolactone can cause hyperkalaemia. However, loop diuretics (e.g. frusemide) and thiazide diuretics (e.g. bendroflumethiazide) are more likely to cause hypokalaemia.

45. **All of the above.** Citrate is commonly used as a preservative in bags of packed red cells. Citrate binds calcium and magnesium, so patients receiving a massive blood transfusion may develop hypocalcaemia and hypomagnesaemia. Haemolysis can occur in bags of packed red cells

during storage, leading to the release of potassium from red blood cells and subsequently causing hyperkalaemia following transfusion. Despite this, hypokalaemia is more common than hyperkalaemia following a massive transfusion. This may be related to a metabolic alkalosis that can occur secondary to citrate metabolism and may also be related to increased potassium uptake by transfused red blood cells that have low levels of intra-cellular potassium.

46. **Calcium gluconate.** An ECG with the appearance of a sine wave is consistent with hyperkalaemia. High potassium levels cause the QRS complex to widen, the T wave to become peaked and the P waves to reduce in size, eventually causing the trace to look like a sine wave. Severe hyperkalaemia should be treated immediately with calcium to prevent arrhythmias. Further treatment is aimed at reducing potassium levels and may include administration of an insulin/dextrose infusion, salbutamol nebulisers, and correction of the cause of the hyperkalaemia.

47. **Para-aortic.** Like the testicles, the ovaries drain to para-aortic lymph nodes.

48. **Decreased urobilinogen excreted in urine.** Bilirubin is converted to urobilinogen in the intestine. Therefore, if the flow of bile into the intestine is obstructed, less urobilinogen will be produced, so less will be excreted. ALT tends to be raised in obstructive jaundice, although alkaline phosphatase is usually raised to a greater extent. Obstructive jaundice causes increased conjugated bilirubin, as conjugation occurs in the liver, before the bile reaches the point of the obstruction.

49. **Loss of skin sensation.** Full-thickness burns are painless due to loss of the sensory nerve endings within the skin. Blisters are a feature of partial thickness burns. First-degree burns affect only the epidermal layer and cause erythema. Partial thickness burns will tend to be moist, whereas full-thickness burns are dry and leathery. In a full-thickness burn, there is hair loss due to destruction of hair follicles, and the ability to sweat is lost due to destruction of sweat glands.

50. **All of the above.** Serum albumin is also included in Child–Pugh scoring. It is graded from A to C and is used to assess prognosis and stratify surgical risk.

MRCS Part A Paper 2

Mock Paper 6

ANSWERS

1. **Hartmann's solution.** Guidelines on fluid resuscitation issued in 2008 suggest crystalloid solutions should be the first line in fluid resuscitation, with Hartmann's solution being the first choice of fluid. (British consensus guidelines on intravenous fluid therapy for adult surgical patients. GIFTASUP; 2009. www.renal.org/pages/media/download_gallery/GIFTASUP%20FINAL_05_01_09.pdf)

2. **Hyperchloraemic acidosis.** Saline 0.9% contains sodium and chloride, which can cause a hyperchloraemia. In turn, this causes a metabolic acidosis with a normal anion gap.

3. **5% dextrose solution.** Dextrose is quickly metabolised once administered, therefore giving continuous volumes of water can result in dilution and hyponatraemia.

4. **30–40 mL/kg/day.** The fluid requirement for the average patient is 30–40 mL/kg/day, approximately 1.5–2.0 L/day.

5. **50–100 mmol/day.** The average 70 kg male requires 50–100 mmol/day of sodium and 40–80 mmol/day of potassium.

6. **3 mg/kg.** The maximum dose of lignocaine is 3 mg/kg and this increases to 7 mg/kg when combined with adrenaline (caution should be exercised when using adrenaline in the distal extremities, e.g. fingers).

7. **2 mg/kg.** This is the maximum dose of bupivacaine that should be administered, whether or not it is combined with adrenaline.

8. **Spinal anaesthesia.** Spinal anaesthetics use a combination of local anaesthetic and opiates such as fentanyl. Depending on what level they are inserted and the level of drug migration through the sub-dural space when the patient is supine, spinals can cause sympathetic blockade resulting in profound hypotension (and even unopposed cardiac parasympathetic stimulation), which can lead to reduced renal perfusion and oliguria.

9. **Opiates.** Opiates are a well-known cause of drowsiness, respiratory depression and confusion in the post-operative patient. It should be noted that drowsiness is a more sensitive indicator of impending opi-ate overdose than RR.

10. **Reduce the background infusion.** When a patient has a PCA, it is advisable to reduce the background infusion in response to drowsi-ness. That way, the patient who is awake can administer a bolus for pain control as and when required.

11. **Airway/C-spine immobilisation.** The ATLS protocol for the management of any trauma follows the A (airway with C-spine immo-bilisation), B (breathing), C (circulation) system.

12. **GCS.** Level of consciousness is assessed by the Glasgow Coma Scale (GCS), different to the Glasgow score, which is used to assess the severity of pancreatitis.

13. **Head CT scan.** Patients often present with head injuries in the context of alcohol consumption and this can mimic neurological symptoms. It is advisable to manage all such patients with caution and follow the NICE guidelines for head CT scans (initial GCS score <15, GCS score <14 after the event, vomiting, amnesia of events, focal neurological deficit) regardless of whether patients have been drinking.

14. **Extradural haemorrhage.** Middle meningeal artery rupture follow-ing trauma to the head causes extradural haemorrhage characterised by a lucid interval after the injury followed by a rapid decline in neu-rological function.

15. **Secondary brain injury.** The management of the head injury patient centres on reducing secondary brain injury from hypoxia and reduced perfusion. CO_2 causes vasodilation of cerebral vessels, therefore

PaCO$_2$ levels should be kept within the range (4–4.5 kPa) to maximise and maintain cerebral perfusion.

16. **Pain.** Compartment syndrome can occur in any fibro-osseous compartment but is probably most common in the leg, particularly after traumatic interventions like intra-medullary nailing. In the conscious patient, pain is the earliest and most reliable sign of increased compartment pressures. Pain on passive stretching should make you very suspicious of a compartment syndrome and instigate prompt action. Compartment pressures can be measured formally with a probe, which is often necessary in unconscious patients.

17. **30 mmHg.** If the difference in pressure between the diastolic BP and the intraosseous compartment pressure is 30 mmHg or less, fasciotomy is indicated.

18. **Split the cast.** If the patient has a backslab or full cast on, this should be split open along its full length; bandages, particularly those that are circumferential and restricting, should also be divided in full.

19. **Volkmann's ischaemic contracture.**

20. **Two incisions.** Fasciotomy to open all four compartments in the leg need only be made by two incisions on either side of the tibia's central tuberosity. The medial incision opens the superficial compartment through which you can access and open the deep compartment. The lateral incision opens the anterior compartment through which you can access and open the lateral compartment. All fascial incisions must be full length.

21. **Closed reduction and fixation with a cast.** How you fix a fracture depends on numerous factors including the type of fracture, what level of function needs to be restored (e.g. dominant versus non-dominant hand) and how well the patient would tolerate a general anaesthetic. In this question, the patient is older with multiple co-morbidities. As the fracture is of the non-dominant hand and she is not an ideal candidate for an anaesthetic, a good closed reduction and fixation with a plaster cast would be appropriate.

22. **Open reduction and internal fixation.** This is a fracture of the dominant hand and there is volar displacement that is unstable – a fracture like this requires plating to ensure the best return of function.

23. **Percutaneous fixation with Kirschner wires.** Supracondylar fractures in children can usually be fixed with Kirschner wires.

24. **Hemiarthroplasty.** Intracapsular neck-of-femur fractures are fixed by cemented or uncemented hemiarthroplasty due to disruption to the blood supply to the head of the femur.

25. **External fixation.** As open fractures carry a significant risk of infection, the insertion of a prosthesis is not advised. As such, these fractures are initially fixed with external fixators to reduce this risk.

26. **Joint aspiration.** Septic arthritis is an orthopaedic emergency that requires prompt evaluation of the patient and joint aspiration for Gram staining as well as microscopy, culture and sensitivities.

27. **Gram stain.** Gram staining should be done within an hour and the presence of bacteria means that the patient should be started on broad-spectrum antibiotics while cultures are pending. Patients at risk of septic arthritis include those with joint replacements and intravenous drug users as well as those with chronic joint disease, rheumatoid arthritis and immunosuppressed patients. Gram-positive aerobes are the most common organisms (*Staphylococcus* and *Streptococcus* species).

28. **Osteoarthritis.** Osteoarthritis is the most common chronic joint disease that particularly affects overweight individuals. Trauma is also a significant risk factor.

29. **Joint-space narrowing and osteophyte formation.** Changes in osteoarthritis that can be observed on X-ray include joint-space narrowing, osteophyte formation, subchondral sclerosis and bone cysts.

30. **Joint-space narrowing and osteopenia.** Rheumatoid arthritis affects predominantly women and can cause carpal tunnel syndrome. It typically affects the small joints of the hand, including the metacarpophalangeal joints (whereas osteoarthritis affects the PIP and DIP joints) and changes observable on X-ray include joint-space narrowing, subluxation, bony erosions and osteopenia.

31. **Varicocele.** This man has renal cell carcinoma, as suggested by his left flank pain, weight loss and haematuria. The insertion of the testicular vein into the renal vein on the left means that people with a renal mass on the left side may present with a left-sided varicocele.

Right-side varicoceles are less common because the right testicular vein inserts directly into the inferior vena cava.

32. **Epididymitis.** The main differential diagnosis here is testicular torsion. However, as the pain has come on gradually and the cremasteric reflex is intact, this is less likely. The patient's recent catheter could be a potential source of infection. Despite the likely diagnosis of epididymo-orchitis, if torsion cannot be ruled out clinically, he may have to undergo scrotal exploration.

33. **Femoral hernia.** A femoral hernia is seen and palpated at the femoral canal, which is situated below and lateral to the pubic tubercle. Femoral hernias are more common in women than men. A cough impulse is not always present.

34. **Hydrocele.** A 'hydrocele' is a collection of serous fluid within the tunica vaginalis. Most hydroceles are painless although some can cause discomfort. They can often be transilluminated. Hydroceles are common in infancy due to patency of the processus vaginalis. Secondary causes that may occur in later life include infection, trauma, tumour and radiotherapy. Changes in the peritoneal fluid may also lead to the development of a hydrocele – for example, in peritoneal dialysis.

35. **Testicular torsion.** The sudden onset of pain is suggestive of torsion, particularly when combined with an absent cremasteric reflex. An abnormal lie would also be suggestive of a diagnosis of testicular torsion. Torsion is most common in adolescents, so this teenager is of an age at which torsion is a likely diagnosis.

36. **Meckel's diverticulitis.** A Meckel's diverticulum is a congenital remnant of the omphalomesenteric duct and found on the anti-mesenteric surface of the small bowel. The appendix is found on the caecum.

37. **Appendices epiploicae.** These are small pouches of fat-filled peritoneum found on the colon and the upper rectum. 'Taeniae coli' are the longitudinally running smooth muscle fibres on the outside of the colon.

38. **Acute cholecystitis.** These symptoms and signs are consistent with acute cholecystitis. The normal liver function tests make cholangitis less likely and a normal level of amylase makes acute pancreatitis unlikely.

39. **Chronic pancreatitis.** These symptoms are of malabsorption, a consequence of chronic pancreatitis, which is associated with long-term alcohol abuse.

40. **Acute cholangitis.** This is a similar presentation to that of cholecystitis, but the presence of pale urine and dark stool (i.e. an obstructive jaundice) make cholangitis a more likely diagnosis.

41. **Intestinal ischaemia.** In a patient who complains of severe pain that is out of proportion to the clinical findings, ischaemia should be suspected. This male has a history of AF, for which he is on aspirin rather than warfarin. It is likely that some thrombus from the heart has embolised and caused the obstruction of blood flow to a section of bowel.

42. **Anal fissure.** Blood on the toilet paper rather than mixed with the stool or in the toilet pan suggests an anal problem. An anal fissure causes pain on defaecation and patients frequently describe it as feeling 'like passing broken glass'.

43. **Inflammatory bowel disease.** The symptoms of altered bowel habit, abdominal pain, and blood and mucus in the stool suggest inflammatory bowel disease, particularly in a young patient who is less likely to have developed other bowel pathologies. Arthralgia is an extra-intestinal feature of inflammatory bowel disease.

44. **Haemorrhoids.** A history of fresh bleeding, noticed on the toilet paper but not mixed in with the stool or in the pan suggests anal bleeding. Pruritus is a common feature of haemorrhoids and there may also be mucous discharge. Haemorrhoids are common in pregnancy. If the patient had a history of chronic constipation, this would also have been suggestive of haemorrhoids.

45. **Peptic ulcer.** An upper GI bleed should be suspected in any patient presenting with heavy, fresh PR bleeding. In this male, a history of steroid use would raise the suspicion of a peptic ulcer, and the presence of epigastric pain and tenderness would support this.

46. **Braided, non-dissolvable suture.** In theory, you may use any suture you like as long as it keeps the drain in place for 24–72 hours, which is the usual time it should stay in the patient. Traditionally, silk is used.

47. **Monofilament, non-dissolvable suture.** A non-dissolvable suture

is necessary to hold the anastomosis, but disruption to lamellar blood flow must be minimised, so a monofilament, which slides easily, is used.

48. **Monofilament, dissolvable suture.** Skin should be closed with an absorbable suture. It will give the tissue support, to enable healing, before dissolving. Monofilament absorbable sutures like Monocryl™ are appropriate, as are braided absorbable suture like Vicryl Rapide™.

49. **Steri-Strip™.** The skin over the tibia is very thin and particularly fragile in older people. Applying Steri-Strips™ reduces skin trauma and spreads the tension over a larger area, while sutures may cut through or cause ischaemia.

50. **Surgical clip.** There are many options for closing the skin of a midline laparotomy, which depend on whether the operation is an emergency or elective procedure, the duration of the procedure and the degree of peritoneal contamination. Surgical clips are advantageous because they are fast to apply (especially in an unwell patient where it is appropriate to limit the operation time to as short as possible), and single clips can be removed to allow superficial collections to drain without needing to open the whole length of the wound.

MRCS Part A Paper 2

Mock Paper 7

ANSWERS

1. **Chest drain insertion, left.** The clinical signs are suggestive of a left-sided haemothorax, which requires drainage using a chest drain.

2. **Bag-mask ventilation.** This patient is not ventilating adequately. She will need a definitive airway in the form of an endotracheal tube. However, as no anaesthetist is available and she is hypoxic, the most appropriate first management step is bag-mask ventilation. She will need a CT scan of her head as part of her ongoing investigation, but it is not currently safe to perform one.

3. **Needle decompression, left thorax.** He has a tension pneumothorax on the left, indicated by hyperresonance and tracheal deviation away from the affected side.

4. **O_2.** O_2 is the most appropriate first management step.

5. **Urgent thoracotomy.** The indication for urgent thoracotomy is drainage of more than 1500 mL immediately on insertion of a chest drain or >200 mL/h.

6. **Allen's test.** An 'Allen's test' involves occluding the radial and ulnar arteries while the patient clenches their fist, then releasing the pressure on the ulnar artery to see if the hand reperfuses. This assesses the collateral flow to the palmar arch via the ulnar artery.

7. **pH 7.35; $PaCO_2$, 4.0; pO_2, 7.8; glucose, 18.0; lactate, 0.8.** This man has symptoms and signs of pancreatitis. As such, his acid–base

status is normal, but he has a raised glucose (secondary to pancreatic dysfunction) and hypoxia.

8. **pH 7.13; PaCO$_2$, 6.5; pO$_2$, 7.9; glucose, 5.9; lactate, 1.2.** This tiring asthmatic will be hypoxic and a concerning sign is rising CO$_2$, as this reflects worsening ability for gas exchange.

9. **pH 6.95; PaCO$_2$, 3.2; pO$_2$, 18.0; glucose, 32.0; lactate, 0.8.** This is a typical new presentation of type 1 diabetes and is suggestive of diabetic ketoacidosis. The ABG sample will characteristically be acidotic with raised glucose and/or reduced CO$_2$ as respiratory compensation.

10. **pH 7.29; PaCO$_2$, 3.2; pO$_2$, 18.4; glucose, 5.6; lactate, 9.2.** This woman's clinical scenario is consistent with ischaemic bowel (due to arterial embolism from AF that is not anticoagulated). This would give her a lactic acidosis.

11. **Atherosclerosis.** Atherosclerosis is the most common cause of carotid artery disease. Stenosis of the carotid artery can impair blood flow, usually to the anterior cerebral circulation, so symptoms tend to involve the face and arms on the contralateral side. Amaurosis fugax (transient visual impairment) and speech impairment can also be features.

12. **Carotid duplex scan.** Carotid artery duplex is the standard imaging performed in patients with neurological symptoms. MRA is more expensive and DSA scans give very accurate information but are invasive and carry a risk of cerebrovascular accident themselves. A CT/MRI brain scan can also be undertaken to look for cerebral infarcts and exclude any other intracranial pathology.

13. **Left carotid endarterectomy.** Symptomatic patients with a carotid artery stenosis of ≥70% should be surgically managed with a carotid endarterectomy of the symptomatic side.

14. **Right carotid endarterectomy.** There is also evidence for asymptomatic patients with a stenosis of 60% or more to be surgically managed.

15. **Anticoagulation.** Patients with newly diagnosed AF, carotid artery stenosis and neurological symptoms should be considered for anticoagulation with warfarin.

16. **Malunion.** 'Malunion' refers to when the bone actually unites but in incorrect alignment. This is usually the result of inadequate reduction initially or inadequate fixation that lets the initial reduction slip into abnormal alignment.

17. **Delayed union.** Delayed union occurs when a healing is slower than usual. This can be the result of patient factors including co-morbidities, malnutrition and steroids.

18. **Hypertrophic non-union.** In intramedullary nailing, removing the proximal and distal locking screws allows loading on the fracture when weight bearing, which often encourages bone healing. 'Non-union' is failure of healing over 3 months; abundant callus formation is 'hypertrophic non-union'.

19. **Avascular necrosis.** Avascular necrosis occurs when a bone's blood supply is compromised so that a portion of the bone is left to necrose – for example, a scaphoid fracture, in which the proximal segment is prone to avascular necrosis because its blood supply runs from distal to proximal.

20. **Atrophic non-union.** Lack of callus formation, as a result of bone resorption, is 'atrophic non-union'. Infection and soft tissue interposition can cause this.

21. **Indirect inguinal hernia.** These arise from weakness in the deep (internal) ring, which allows intra-abdominal structures to herniate through the deep ring, along the inguinal canal and through the superficial (external) ring. Direct inguinal hernias arise from a defect in the abdominal wall behind the superficial ring. Therefore, if a hernia is reduced and the internal ring is covered, a direct hernia will still protrude on coughing while an indirect hernia will not.

22. **Indirect inguinal hernia.** Indirect inguinal hernia sacs arise lateral to the inferior epigastric artery at operation and direct inguinal hernia sacs run medially.

23. **Femoral hernia.** Femoral hernias lie inferior and medial to the pubic tubercle. They are more common in women.

24. **Testicular artery.** Testicular atrophy may result from damage to the testicular artery at the time of hernia repair.

25. **Ilioinguinal nerve.** The ilioinguinal nerve supplies the skin of the

scrotum and medial thigh (in men) and the mons pubis and labia (in women).

26. **Spinal shock.** 'Spinal shock' is spinal cord injury resulting in neurological impairment below the level of the injury.

27. **Neurogenic shock.** 'Neurogenic shock' refers to autonomic dysfunction and its effects below the level of the spinal cord injury.

28. **C-spine immobilisation.** Following any trauma, ATLS protocol should be followed: A (airway) plus C-spine immobilisation, B (breathing) and C (circulation). C-spine immobilisation has three parts: stiff neck collar, blocks either side of the head, which are strapped to the patient, and a board beneath their head.

29. **Stable fracture.** Unilateral facet dislocations are generally considered stable.

30. **CT scan of the spine.** Imaging of the spine following trauma should start with plain radiographs. Following this, as CT shows good bony pathology, it is useful for fracture assessment post trauma. MRI shows good soft tissue pathology and is used subsequently to assess nerve involvement.

31. **Unintentional weight loss >10% in 3–6 months.** 'Malnutrition' is defined by NICE as a BMI <18.5, unintentional weight loss >10% in the last 3–6 months or a BMI <20 with unintentional weight loss >5% within 3–6 months. (National Institute for Health and Clinical Excellence. Nutrition Support in Adults; oral nutrition support, enteral tube feeding and parenteral nutrition: NICE guideline 32. London: NIHCE; 2006. www.nice.org.uk/guidance/CG32)

32. **Enteral.** Enteral feeding – either by encouraged oral intake and supplementation or formal enteral feeding via a NG/NJ/PEG/PEJ tube – is the preferred method of nutritional support.

33. **Prevent bacterial translocation.** The gut mucosa deteriorates without luminal nutrients to absorb; consequently, the barrier is broken down, allowing gut organisms and endotoxins to pass across.

34. **Small bowel fistula.** Enteral feeds are contraindicated in patients with small bowel fistula and high-output proximal stoma in which enteral feeds will drive secretions. In addition, in cases of impaired

gastric motility, delivering large-volume enteral feeds into the stomach increases a patient's aspiration risk.

35. **Percutaneous gastrostomy.** If enteral feeds are required for longer than 6 weeks, patients should be considered for PEG/PEJ tube insertion, as NG tubes are uncomfortable for patients and cause irritation in the long-term.

36. **4 mL.** The maximum dose of plain bupivacaine is 2 mg/kg; that is, 20 mg for this child. Bupivacaine 0.5% contains 5 mg/mL, thus you may use up to 4 mL.

37. **42 mL.** The maximum dose of plain lignocaine is 3 mg/kg and 7 mg/kg with adrenaline; that is, 420 mg for a 60 kg patient. Lignocaine 1% contains 10 mg/mL, so you may use up to 42 mL.

38. **12 mL.** An 80 kg male may have $3 \times 80 = 240$ mg of plain lignocaine. Lignocaine 2% contains 20 mg/mL, therefore up to 12 mL may be used.

39. **0.5% bupivacaine.** Plain local anaesthetic should be used on appendages with end arteries, such as the fingers or the penis. If local anaesthetic containing adrenaline is used, the end artery may spasm, risking ischaemia of the extremity.

40. **Intralipid®.** Intralipid® is the antidote for local-anaesthetic toxicity. As such, it is important to know where is it kept in your department before administering local anaesthetic.

41. **Sensitivity.** 'Sensitivity' refers to the proportion of those who have the disease who are correctly identified as having the disease by the test in question; that is, true positives/(true positives + false negatives).

42. **Negative predictive value.** 'Negative predictive value' refers to the proportion of those who the test identifies as negative who do not have the disease in reality; that is, true negatives/(true negatives + false negatives). 'Positive predictive value' is the proportion of those who the test identifies as positive who really do have the disease; that is, true positives/(true positives + false positives).

43. **Specificity.** This refers to the proportion of those without the disease who are correctly identified as being disease-free.

44. **Relative risk.** The 'relative risk' is the number of individuals who

develop the disease in group 1 divided by the number who develop the disease in group 2. It compares proportions/percentages.

45. **Incidence.** 'Incidence' is the number of new cases over a specified period, while 'prevalence' is the number of cases identified in a population at a single time point.

46. **Bladder outlet obstruction.** An enlarged prostate, causing bladder outflow obstruction, is very likely to bleed.

47. **Transitional cell carcinoma of the bladder.** Smoking is the biggest independent risk factor for transitional cell carcinoma. Patients with similar presentations should be appropriately investigated.

48. **Bladder outlet obstruction.** Bladder outlet obstruction results in residual volumes post voiding, which predisposes to infection.

49. **Renal stones.** Stones are a cause of painful haematuria and patients with an ileal conduit are at increased risk of stone formation.

50. **Prostatitis.** Prostatic infections will cause pain and sometimes bleeding.

MRCS Part A Paper 2

Mock Paper 8

ANSWERS

1. **Hashimoto's thyroiditis.** This patient has the symptoms of hypothyroidism. Hashimoto's will present with a goitre and hypothyroidism.

2. **Graves' disease.** Graves' will present with a goitre and either euthyroidism or hyperthyroidism. This patient has the symptoms of thyrotoxicosis.

3. **Anaplastic carcinoma.** The cragginess of the mass and weight loss are suggestive of malignancy and the hoarse voice suggests infiltration of the recurrent laryngeal nerve. Most thyroid cancers do not invade locally, but anaplastic carcinomas are aggressive, invade locally and generate systemic features of malignancy.

4. **Thyroid lobectomy.** Follicular adenoma is difficult to distinguish from follicular carcinoma on FNA, as the cells look the same cytologically. It is their histological architecture that distinguishes the two pathologies. A follicular adenoma is benign and may be treated with a thyroid lobectomy (to reduce the chance of hypocalcaemia resulting from damage to the parathyroid glands, which is higher in a total thyroidectomy).

5. **Total thyroidectomy.** Follicular carcinomas must be treated with a total thyroidectomy, as they are malignant.

6. **Intussusception.** 'Intussusception' is the telescoping of bowel into itself. It presents with pain, which is usually intermittent due to the colicky contraction of the telescoped bowel. The rectal bleeding may

be described as looking like redcurrant jelly and this, together with a sausage-shaped abdominal mass, is typical of intussusception.

7. **Mesenteric adenitis.** The preceding viral illness with generalised lymphadenopathy and persistent fever make the aetiology of this patient's abdominal pain most likely to be due to mesenteric adenitis. Its variability, as opposed to localisation to the right iliac fossa, also distinguishes it from appendicitis.

8. **Pyloric stenosis.** Pyloric stenosis is characterised by projectile vomiting, starting between 1 week and 5 months of age. It is rare in children older than 6 months. It normally presents at ~3 weeks of age and is more common in male children. A mass may sometimes be palpable in the epigastrium.

9. **Appendicitis.** The migratory nature of the pain and associated anorexia are characteristic of appendicitis, along with the low-grade temperature and localised peritonism.

10. **Gastroschisis.** 'Gastroschisis' is the congenital absence of the abdominal wall at the midline due to failure of fusion of the two lateral components in utero. It is distinguished from exomphalos by the absence of a sac/overlying peritoneum.

11. **Erect chest X-ray.** This female may have a perforated peptic ulcer secondary to NSAID use. It is important to look for air under the diaphragm.

12. **Mesenteric angiogram.** This patient has ongoing GI bleeding and is shocked despite resuscitation. Ideally, this patient should go to theatre for operative intervention. However, her multiple co-morbidities and recent myocardial infarction mean that her chances of surviving an anaesthetic are relatively small. A mesenteric angiogram would allow localisation of the source of bleeding, as well as enable therapeutic intervention without the need for an anaesthetic.

13. **Abdominal/pelvic USS.** In this age group, intermittent severe abdominal pain with obstructive symptoms suggests a possible diagnosis of intussusception. A USS should be obtained, preferably during a painful episode, to rule out this condition.

14. **Colonoscopy.** This male requires a colonoscopy to investigate his

symptoms. In this age group, a persistent change in bowel habit asso-ciated with rectal bleeding may indicate bowel cancer.

15. **Abdominal X-ray.** The symptoms of vomiting, constipation, abdom-inal pain and distension are highly suggestive of bowel obstruction. It is likely that this male will require a CT scan to determine the aetiol-ogy. However, the initial investigation should be an abdominal X-ray to determine whether there are dilated loops of bowel and whether there is an obvious transition point between dilated bowel and col-lapsed bowel.

16. **Cardiogenic shock.** A raised jugular venous pulse with bibasal crackles suggest fluid overload. The pallor and sweatiness may be secondary to an acute cardiac event.

17. **Hypovolaemic shock.** This patient is shocked post-operatively, with tachycardia, hypotension and oliguria. The most likely cause is hypovolaemia.

18. **Septic shock.** This child is tachycardic and febrile, fulfilling two of the four SIRS criteria. In addition, he has a clinical source of infec-tion (in the form of a positive urine dipstick). Therefore, he has septic shock.

19. **SIRS.** SIRS requires the presence of two or more of: HR >90 bpm, T <36.0°C or >38.0°C, RR >20 breaths/min, and WCC <4 × 10^9/L or >12 × 10^9/L. SIRS + clinical source of infection = sepsis. However, this man's most likely diagnosis is pancreatitis and his physiological derangement is secondary to SIRS, without any evidence of a clinical source of infection.

20. **Anaphylactic shock.** This patient is shocked following administra-tion of a known sensitising agent.

21. **LMWH only.** This patient requires prophylaxis, but TED® stock-ings are contraindicated by his diabetic neuropathy.

22. **None.** LMWH is contraindicated preoperatively when spinal or epidural anaesthesia is planned and in spinal, neuro and ophthalmic surgery due to the bleeding risk. He cannot wear TED® stockings due to his neuropathy.

23. **TED® stockings and LMWH.** This patient requires prophylaxis

and, providing her renal function is normal, has no contraindications to LMWH or TED® stockings.

24. **TED® stockings and LMWH.** This patient requires prophylaxis and has no contraindications to LMWH or TED® stockings.

25. **LMWH and compression pumps.** In patients with lymphoedema, it will be difficult to fit TED® stockings onto large legs, so compression pumps should be used.

26. **Chronic venous insufficiency.** Venous hypertension causes extravasation of red blood cells that results in haemosiderin deposits (brown staining) and fibrin deposition from the local inflammatory reaction that ensues (lipodermatosclerosis and eventual shrinking of the lower part of the leg, producing the inverted champagne bottle shape).

27. **Chronic venous insufficiency.** The 'gaiter' region of the leg is the medial aspect of the lower leg and is classically (although not always) the site of venous ulceration.

28. **Deep vein thrombosis.** Deep vein thrombosis must be excluded prior to any varicose vein operation to ensure that the superficial system is not the only venous drainage method for that limb before it is stripped out.

29. **Four-layer compression bandaging.** Four-layer compression bandages are the treatment for venous ulcers provided the patient has good arterial supply to the leg. The 'ABPI' is the ratio of ankle to brachial pressure as measured by a sphygmomanometer. A ratio of 1.0 denotes no arterial disease.

30. **Marjolin's ulcer.** Any ulceration failing to heal should be biopsied to look for evidence of cancer. Marjolin's ulcer is a squamous-cell carcinoma that can arise from venous ulcers.

31. **Closed reduction and cast.** When there is obvious joint deformity and neurovascular compromise, the fracture should be immediately reduced and immobilised in alignment with a backslab or brace. While this is true for all fractures, it is particularly important for ankle fractures to reduce the swelling that ensues – many ankle-fracture open reduction internal fixations are delayed due to excessive swelling resulting in difficulties with skin closure after the operation. For this reason, it is also essential to elevate the limb as soon as possible.

32. **Weber B.** Distal fibula fractures are classified as Weber A when they are below the level of the syndesmosis, Weber B at the level of the syndesmosis and Weber C above the level of the syndesmosis. The syndesmosis provides the necessary tough ligamentous stability to the ankle mortise joint to ensure function.

33. **Open reduction and internal fixation.** As injuries at or above the syndesmosis imply damage to the ligamentous stability, these are treated more aggressively with open reduction and internal fixation rather than simple casting. 'Diastasis of the syndesmosis' is widening or separation that occurs following high-energy injuries. Energy starts at the medial side of the ankle joint and will travel the full length of the interosseous membrane between the fibula and tibia. Therefore, in your clinical assessment, you must ensure that you have looked for possible fractures along that energy line. This often means obtaining a knee X-ray.

34. **Maisonneuve fracture.** A 'Maisonneuve fracture' is a fracture of the proximal fibula, which occurs with high-energy fractures of the medial malleolus and disruption of the syndesmosis.

35. **AP, lateral and mortise plain films.** X-rays of the ankle joint must include a mortise view. All orthopaedic assessments should include AP and lateral views of the joint above and below the injury site.

36. **Cystic duct.** The cystic duct forms the lateral border of the triangle, the common hepatic duct forms the medial border and the inferior edge of the liver forms the superior border.

37. **Mascagni's node.** The only structure, other than cystic artery, contained *within* Calot's triangle is Mascagni's node, the lymph node associated with the gallbladder. It may be enlarged in cholecystitis or cholangitis.

38. **Pringle's manoeuvre.** 'Pringle's manoeuvre' is the compression of the hepatoduodenal ligament (which contains the hepatic artery and portal vein), either between your finger and thumb or with a haemo-static clamp, to control bleeding from the liver.

39. **Falciform ligament.** The falciform ligament lies anterior to the liver, between the left and right lobes. It is seen at laparoscopic cholecystectomy and the epigastric port is sited just lateral to it.

The cardiac ligament is on the superior surface of the liver and not seen.

40. **Common bile duct.** The cystic duct, along with the cystic artery, is clipped and divided at laparoscopic cholecystectomy. However, if the common bile duct is accidentally damaged, bile may leak into the peritoneum.

41. **Posterior hip dislocation.** Following total hip replacement in which the joint capsule and ligaments are divided, joint stability is less than that of a native hip joint. This is more so in certain surgical approaches to the hip but generally patients are advised not to sit on low chairs, as there is a risk of joint dislocation after 90 degrees of hip flexion. Posterior hip dislocation is common with prostheses.

42. **Posterior hip dislocation.** Posterior hip dislocation (usually with an associated fracture) may also occur in road traffic accidents as a result of the front seat passenger's knees being compressed against the dashboard.

43. **Femoral nerve.** All hip dislocations in adults require considerable force, thus are often associated with acetabular fractures, head-of-femur fractures and nerve injuries (the sciatic nerve in posterior dislocations and the femoral nerve in anterior dislocations).

44. **Pubic ramus fracture.** Pubic ramus fractures are also common in older patients presenting to A&E after a fall. There is often marked tenderness over the groin and pain on weight bearing.

45. **AP, lateral and Judet view plain films.** Pelvic fractures can be seen best with proper imaging of the pelvis on AP, lateral and Judet view plain films.

46. **Pyelonephritis.** As the urine dipstick result is positive for nitrites (though not leucocytes), the patient has flank pain and is pyrexial, pyelonephritis is the most likely diagnosis.

47. **Diabetic ketoacidosis.** Diabetic ketoacidosis may present with abdominal pain and vomiting, as well as polyuria. It is important to pay attention to the urine dipstick, which in this case is positive for ketones and glucose.

48. **Renal colic.** Severe, colicky pain (often requiring morphine), with

either visible or invisible haematuria is typical of renal colic. Diabetic ketoacidosis would result in glycosuria and ketonuria.

49. **Abdominal aortic aneurysm rupture.** Abdominal aortic aneurysms occur in 5% of men over the age of 55. A ruptured aneurysm may mimic renal colic but needs to be excluded, especially with a negative urine dipstick and when haemodynamically unstable.

50. **Appendicitis.** The history of migratory right iliac fossa pain with a fever is typical of appendicitis.

MRCS Part A Paper 2

Mock Paper 9

ANSWERS

1. **Reactive lymph node.** The preceding coryzal symptoms and the fact that a number of lumps are palpable make a reactive lymph node most likely.

2. **Sebaceous cyst.** Sebaceous cysts arise within the dermis. They may become intermittently infected (as in this scenario). Characteristically, they have a central punctum.

3. **Thyroglossal cyst.** A 'thyroglossal cyst' is a congenital remnant of the thyroglossal tract that is formed as the thyroid descends from the base of the tongue during embryological development. It therefore moves on swallowing and tongue protrusion.

4. **Branchial cyst.** These are remnants of the branchial clefts (most commonly the second) and are found in the anterior triangle of the neck. They are usually asymptomatic but may become infected, meriting their excision.

5. **Cystic hygroma.** A 'cystic hygroma' is a congenital lymphangioma associated with chromosomal abnormalities. It occurs in the posterior triangle of the neck, most commonly the left.

6. **3.** The GCS (which has a minimum score of 3 and maximum of 15), assesses consciousness level based on the patient's *best* eye opening, motor response and verbal response, as illustrated in the following table.

	Eye opening		Best verbal response		Best motor response
4	Spontaneous	5	Orientated	6	Obeys commands
3	To speech	4	Confused	5	Localises pain
2	To pain	3	Inappropriate words	4	Normal flexion to pain
1	None	2	Incomprehensible sounds	3	Abnormal flexion to pain
		1	None	2	Extension to pain
				1	None

7. **10.** The motor component of the GCS includes the patient's *best* motor response (i.e. in this case, withdrawing from rather than flexing to pain). Eye opening = 3, best verbal response = 2, best motor response = 5.

8. **11**

9. **4**

10. **14**

11. **Anterior cruciate ligament.** Anterior cruciate ligament tears are common and sustained from twisting injuries when the knee is in slight flexion (hence, these are a common skiing injury). The clinical history is immediate acute swelling, which is usually haemarthrosis from the ruptured ligament. Patients then report instability in the knee caused by the tibia sliding forwards on weight bearing in flexion.

12. **Lachman's test.** Lachman's test is described in the question. Along with the anterior draw test, it assesses anterior cruciate ligament stability.

13. **Medial meniscal injury.** Meniscal injuries are common (medial more so than lateral), and joint line tenderness, combined with a feeling of instability, locking or clicking, and delayed swelling are classical signs. They are sustained in sports in which there is a sudden change in direction with weight load on the knee joint.

14. **Medial collateral ligament.** As the medial meniscus is attached to the medial collateral ligament, this must also be assessed for injury. McMurray's test assesses meniscal injuries but is poorly tolerated by patients, so not often performed.

15. **Diagnostic arthroscopy and/or meniscectomy.** A suspected meniscal injury warrants diagnostic arthroscopy and/or proceeding to treatment (meniscectomy) of the meniscal injury. An arthroscopic washout is used in septic arthritis.

16. **Enteral feeding via NG tube.** Surgical patients are at risk of becoming malnourished once they have had no or minimal oral intake for 5 days or more. This is especially significant in critical illness when the body is in a catabolic state. When appropriate, enteral feeding is the preferred method, initially via NG tube.

17. **Parenteral feeding via central line.** Patients with a gut <300 cm generally require TPN, at least temporarily, until enteral feeds are established. A short gut of <100 cm usually renders the patient TPN dependent.

18. **Parenteral feeding via central line.** Patients at high risk of post-operative ileus – for example, those having had major abdominal surgery and with intra-abdominal sepsis – should have their nutritional requirements carefully assessed. As this patient is still on the ICU with respiratory support, it would be advisable to start and continue TPN until the ileus resolves.

19. **Re-feeding syndrome.** Re-feeding syndrome is not common but should be guarded against in patients on TPN. Daily electrolyte measurements, including of magnesium and phosphate, are required. Symptoms include confusion and muscle weakness.

20. **Line sepsis.** A pancreatic pseudocyst is a relative contraindication for enteral feeding, as it may exacerbate pain and cause gastric outlet obstruction. When TPN is used, it must be given via central access via a dedicated line not used for anything else, such as blood taking or IV fluids. The groin should be avoided as a site for central access and TPN administration to reduce the risk of line sepsis.

21. **Anterior dislocation.** Anterior shoulder dislocations are common sporting injuries that result from falling on an outstretched arm. The normal contour of the shoulder is lost, as the humeral head sits on the anterior chest wall beneath the clavicle.

22. **Posterior dislocation.** A posterior dislocation of the shoulder is much less common than an anterior dislocation and typically occurs

post epileptic seizure or in patients who have sustained an electric shock. However, it can occur in patients who are violently assaulted. On X-ray, the light bulb sign is indicative of this dislocation.

23. **Axillary nerve function.**

24. **Axillary nerve function.** When assessing a patient with a shoulder dislocation, the axillary nerve function must always be assessed before and after a closed reduction (by assessing sensation over the regimental badge area).

25. **Hill–Sachs lesion.** Patients who suffer recurrent dislocations often sustain bony lesions to the humeral head during anterior dislocation. These are called 'Hill–Sachs lesions'. 'Bankart lesions' are inferior tears of the glenoid labrum, although bony Bankart lesions involving fractures of the glenoid itself can also occur.

26. **Gastric outlet obstruction.** This patient presents with vomiting and his blood gas sample shows a hypokalaemic and hypochloraemic metabolic alkalosis.

27. **Ischaemic bowel.** This patient presents with abdominal pain and a risk factor for ischaemic bowel. Her blood gas sample shows metabolic acidosis (with respiratory compensation) with a high lactate suggestive of ischaemic tissue (in this case, of the gut).

28. **Pulmonary embolism.** This patient presents with shortness of breath and malignancy (a risk factor for deep vein thrombosis/pulmonary embolism). Her blood gas sample shows hypoxia. Investigation for a pulmonary embolism is warranted.

29. **Anxiety.** This patient presents with symptoms suggestive of anxiety (shortness of breath and circumoral tingling). Her blood gas sample shows a respiratory alkalosis suggesting she is hyperventilating.

30. **Diabetic ketoacidosis.** This patient presents with a failing pancreas transplant. His blood gas sample shows a metabolic acidosis, hyperkalaemia and hyperglycaemia. Urinalysis showing ketonuria would confirm the diagnosis of diabetic ketoacidosis.

31. **Hashimoto's thyroiditis.** Anti-thyroid peroxidase is found in serum in Hashimoto's thyroiditis.

32. **Atrophic gastritis.** Atrophic gastritis is caused by antibody destruction of parietal cells in the stomach. This leads to diminished intrinsic

factor and pernicious anaemia usually follows. However, antibodies to intrinsic factor are causative in pernicious anaemia (intrinsic factor impairs the absorption of vitamin B12 and subsequently causes megaloblastic macrocytic anaemia).

33. **Goodpasture's syndrome.** Goodpasture's syndrome is a type II hypersensitivity reaction to the antigen glomerular basement membrane found in the lungs and kidneys. It causes bleeding and renal failure.

34. **Myasthenia gravis.** In this autoimmune condition, antibodies to acetylcholine receptors block the action of the neurotransmitter acetylcholine, causing fatigable weakness. Myasthenia gravis is managed with acetylcholinesterase inhibitors.

35. **Scleroderma.** Rheumatoid arthritis is diagnosed by the presence of rheumatoid factor in serum. Patients with systemic lupus erythematosus can have circulating anti-double stranded DNA antibodies, anti-phospholipid antibodies (lupus anticoagulant) and anti-cardiolipin antibodies.

36. **Hypercalcaemia.** Hypercalcaemia occurs as part of a paraneoplastic syndrome and produces non-specific symptoms including abdominal pain, malaise, constipation and cognitive change.

37. **Anastomotic leak.** Anastomotic leaks can present themselves at any time and, in this case, you should be mindful to check the creatinine of the serous fluid to determine if it is a urine leak.

38. **Intra-abdominal collection.** A post-operative intra-abdominal collection is not uncommon and you should be alert for signs of one developing, including a SIRS response, rising WCC/CRP level or symptoms such as diarrhoea and abdominal pain.

39. **Ileus.** Patients can develop an ileus after any sort of abdominal operation. Typically, they will complain of abdominal discomfort/bloating and have not opened their bowels, although they may be passing flatus. High NG output is a consequence of ileus.

40. **Abdominal compartment syndrome.** After a delayed period with a laparostomy, the rectus muscles diverge and are often difficult to close. Consequently, they can be very tight and you should cautiously

monitor the patient (particularly if they are still intubated on the ITU) for signs of abdominal compartment syndrome.

41. **Gentamicin.** Gentamicin may cause sensorineural hearing loss and renal toxicity.

42. **Steroid.** Steroids may cause acne and fluid retention.

43. **Rifampicin.** Rifampicin may cause jaundice and yellow discoloration of all body fluids (including urine and tears).

44. **Steroid.** Steroids may also cause a proximal myopathy.

45. **Heparin.** Heparin may cause a heparin-induced thrombocytopenia and patients receiving LMWH should also have their platelet levels monitored.

46. **Incision for lateral approach to hip.**

47. **Oblique incision for inguinal hernia repair.**

48. **Midline raphe incision for testicular exploration.**

49. **Lumbar puncture.**

50. **Incision for carpal tunnel decompression.**

MRCS Part A Paper 2

Mock Paper 10

ANSWERS

1. **Fibroadenoma.** In this age group, the majority of breast lumps are benign. Fibroadenomas are typically smooth, firm and mobile lumps nicknamed 'breast mice' due to their mobility.

2. **Mammography and FNA.** Every female presenting to the breast clinic should undergo triple assessment in the form of clinical assessment, imaging (USS or mammography) and tissue sampling (FNA or core biopsy). Women under the age of 35 should have a USS rather than mammography, as their denser breasts make mammography difficult to interpret.

3. **Mastectomy.** While it is right to focus on breast-preserving surgery, a 5 cm carcinoma (requiring a 7 cm excision) in a slim female would result in a poor oncological and aesthetic result compared with mastectomy with reconstruction.

4. **Reassurance.** Bilateral cyclical breast pain is common. However, the patient should be assessed clinically for any masses and advised on regular breast self-examination.

5. **USS and FNA.** This is most likely a breast cyst, which should be imaged and aspirated. If clear, greenish fluid is aspirated with no blood and the lump completely resolves after aspiration, no further investigation is needed. However, if there is a solid component to the lump, it should be sampled, and if there is a bloodstained aspirate, it should be sent for cytological analysis.

6. **Cannulated screws.** It is common for older people with neck-of-femur fractures to present to A&E. There are many different ways to fix these, depending on where the fracture is and whether the blood supply to the head of the femur (running through the retinacular arteries in the hip joint capsule and diaphyseal vessels from distal to proximal) has been affected. Cannulation screws are appropriate when the fracture is intracapsular, undisplaced and impacted.

7. **Proximal femoral nail.** Proximal femoral nailing works best when the fracture is below the trochanteric line.

8. **Dynamic hip screw.** Intracapsular fractures are fixed with hemiarthroplasty and extracapsular fractures by dynamic hip screw.

9. **Neurovascular status of the limb.** A mandatory part of your clinical assessment is the neurovascular status of the limb.

10. **Assess fitness for surgery.** Prior to any management decision, patients must be assessed for their pre-morbid level of function and fitness for surgery.

11. **Infected prosthesis.**

12. **Reperfusion injury.**

13. **Lactate >1.2 mmol/L.** 'Organ dysfunction' is defined in the cardiovascular system as lactate >1.2 mmol/L, in the respiratory system as PaO_2 <9.3 kPa, in the renal system as a urine output <120 mL over 4 hours and in the CNS as a GCS score <15 when patient is not sedated.

14. **Soft tissue infection.**

15. **Refractory hypotension.** 'Systemic inflammatory response' is defined as two or more of the following: pyrexia >38°C/hypothermia <35°C, tachycardia HR>90 bpm, tachypnoea RR>20, WCC >12× 10^9/L/<4, acutely altered mental state, blood glucose >6.6 mmol/L (non-diabetics). 'Sepsis' is the presence of SIRS and a proven infection source. 'Severe sepsis' requires a confirmed infection with dysfunction in one or more organs. 'Sepsis syndrome' occurs when no infection is confirmed but organ dysfunction is present. This is defined in the cardiovascular system as lactate >1.2 mmol/L, in the respiratory system as PaO_2 <9.3 kPa, in the renal system as a urine output <120 mL over 4 hours and in the CNS as a GCS score <15 when the patient is not

sedated. 'Septic shock' is when there is organ dysfunction, infection and refractory hypotension.

16. **Monteggia fracture.** A 'Monteggia fracture' is a fracture of the ulnar shaft (usually the proximal third) and displacement of the head of the radius.

17. **Galeazzi fracture.** A 'Galeazzi fracture' is more distal than a Monteggia, affecting the radius shaft with dislocation of the distal radioulnar joint.

18. **Tetanus status.** All patients with open fractures should have their tetanus status assessed and clearly documented in their notes. Patients should be vaccinated immediately if there is any doubt as to their status.

19. **Osteoarthritis.** Patients with intra-articular fractures are at risk of long-term osteoarthritis, even if they have undergone fixation.

20. **Complex regional pain syndrome.** A 'Barton's fracture' of the distal radius is a fracture that has volar displacement in which the fracture extends down into the joint line. It is an unstable fracture that should be fixed by open reduction and internal fixation. Patients should be informed of 'complex regional pain syndrome', in which the hand becomes swollen and painful for an indeterminate time after surgical intervention. This syndrome is a cause of great morbidity to those patients who suffer from it, thus it is wise to counsel your patients before the operation.

21. **Midline incision for laparotomy.**

22. **Neck incision for tracheotomy.**

23. **Neck incision for cricothyroidotomy.**

24. **Lanz incision for appendicectomy.**

25. **Lumbar incision for nerve root decompression.**

26. **Conjunctivitis.** Inflammation of the conjunctival layer is commonly due to infection.

27. **Episcleritis.** Episcleritis is a less serious condition that seldom progresses to the more serious scleritis.

28. **Keratitis.** Contact-lens wearers have to be careful not to scar the cornea, which occurs usually as a result of infection.

29. **Acute angle glaucoma.** Acute angle glaucoma is a sight-threatening emergency.

30. **Subconjunctival haemorrhage.** Severe coughing can produce such pressure that small friable blood vessels in the conjunctiva can burst.

31. **Congenital bicuspid valve.** A congenitally bicuspid aortic valve is the most common cause of *early* onset aortic stenosis in the United Kingdom. Age-related aortic sclerosis is the most common cause of aortic stenosis overall. Rheumatic fever is rare in the United Kingdom and the resultant valve disease typically presents with a childhood history of rheumatic fever.

32. **Narrow pulse pressure.** A narrow pulse pressure (as a result of relative systolic hypotension) and a slow-rising pulse are clinical signs of aortic stenosis.

33. **Collapsing pulse.** A diastolic murmur that radiates to the carotids is consistent with aortic regurgitation, which will be associated with a collapsing pulse.

34. **Flow murmur.** Pregnancy is a hyperdynamic state that often results in an audible flow murmur.

35. **Mitral regurgitation.** A pansystolic murmur that radiates to the patient's apex and is displaced laterally and inferiorly is a characteristic mitral regurgitation murmur.

36. *Cytomegalovirus.*

37. *Staphylococcus epidermidis.*

38. *Pseudomonas aeruginosa.*

39. *Streptococcus pneumoniae.*

40. *Streptococcus pyogenes.*

41. **Acute cholecystitis.** A female in this age group with a history of intermittent abdominal pain after meals suggests biliary colic. However, the fact that she is also febrile makes cholecystitis the most likely diagnosis. Post-prandial pain may also be associated with a peptic ulcer, but this pain is usually immediate rather than delayed.

42. **Ureteric colic.** The colicky nature of this patient's pain (his restlessness and inability to get comfortable, which are typical of colic) and non-visible haematuria are characteristic of renal colic.

43. **Diverticulitis.** Diverticular disease characteristically affects the left colon and tends to be exacerbated by constipation. It may present either as diverticulitis (as in this case) or with rectal bleeding.

44. **Ruptured aortic aneurysm.** This man has a standard history of a ruptured aortic aneurysm on a background of vascular risk factors (age, sex and history of previous vascular problems) and is haemodynamically unstable. As such, the most important diagnosis to consider is that of a ruptured abdominal aortic aneurysm.

45. **Duodenal ulcer.** Steroids and NSAIDs may cause peptic ulcer disease. Epigastric pain is the common clinical presentation, which may be exacerbated or relieved by eating, belching and bloating.

46. **No consent required.** As this is an immediately life-saving procedure, it is performed in the patient's best interests (in the absence of an advanced directive stating otherwise).

47. **Consent Form 1.** A Consent Form 1 is signed by the patient who will be undergoing the procedure, provided they have capacity to give or withhold consent.

48. **Consent Form 2.** A Consent Form 2 is signed by the parent or legal guardian of a child undergoing a procedure. In cases of older children who disagree with their parents' wishes, their competence (Gillick/Fraser) should be assessed to determine whether they are able to give consent themselves.

49. **Consent Form 4.** A Consent Form 4 is used when a patient is unable to consent to a procedure themselves but the procedure is deemed to be in their best interests. This may be either temporary (for example, when the patient is unconscious and unlikely to regain consciousness in time to give consent) or permanent (as in this scenario).

50. **Verbal consent.** Verbal consent is sufficient for procedures involving no impairment of consciousness (i.e. anaesthesia or sedation), such as blood tests or the reduction of a fracture in A&E.

Index

CPD with Radcliffe

You can now use a selection of our books to achieve CPD (Continuing Professional Development) points through directed reading.

We provide a free online form and downloadable certificate for your appraisal portfolio. Look for the CPD logo and register with us at: www.radcliffehealth.com/cpd

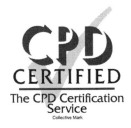